PHARMACOLOGICAL
EXPERIMENTS ON
INTACT PREPARATIONS

PHARMACOLOGICAL EXPERIMENTS ON INTACT PREPARATIONS

The Staff of the
Department of Pharmacology
University of Edinburgh

and

L. J. McLeod,
M.Sc., M.P.S., A.R.A.C.I.
School of Pharmacy, Hobart Technical College, Tasmania

E. & S. LIVINGSTONE
EDINBURGH AND LONDON
1970

ISBN 0 443 00731 4

Printed in Great Britain

CONTENTS

Chapter I

GENERAL METHODS

INTRODUCTION

This book is intended to be a companion to *Pharmacological Experiments on Isolated Preparations*. There are, however, big differences between the two types of experiment. The effects of a drug in a whole animal are complicated by the possibility that what is observed is the consequence of the drug acting at many sites at once. This is very important, for example, when considering the effects of drugs on the blood-pressure, where the change in pressure observed is the consequence of many actions, which may even oppose each other. The experiments are also complicated because the effect produced will depend partly on how the drug is administered, whether it reaches its sites of action immediately or only slowly over a long period. The action of the body on the drug is also important. The effects observed will depend upon the rate of excretion and metabolism of the drug and may be quite different from those observed with isolated preparations, where the drug is added in a known concentration at a known time to a small piece of tissue and washed out at a known time. The effects of suxamethonium and decamethonium on the isolated rat diaphragm preparation, for instance, are virtually indistinguishable but on an intact preparation, such as the cat tibialis (p. 37), the effects are quite different. Intact preparations have the great advantage that they indicate the likely clinical effects of a drug much better than isolated preparations but they have the disadvantage that it may be much more difficult to work out how the drug is acting. Clearly both types of experiment are necessary.

For practical reasons, however, experiments with intact preparations are much more difficult to organize for students. They usually take a lot of time. Many preparations involve lengthy dissection and the time available for testing drugs is limited. As the drugs cannot be 'washed out', the use of too big a dose may involve waiting, perhaps for as long as an hour, while the effects wear off. The experiments are more expensive than those with isolated preparations, require a greater manual skill, and it is often difficult to arrange for students to see what is going on satisfactorily. In Britain experiments on living animals come under Home Office control and must only be performed by people who have the necessary licence and certificates (p. 31). For all these reasons this book involves more description of the methods for setting up preparations than its companion and a smaller number of actual experiments with drugs. It is hoped, however, that these descriptions will be useful because the preparations can be used for a variety of experiments both for teaching and research.

Some experiments are included which involve human subjects. These do not come under the Cruelty to Animals Act, 1876, but the legal and ethical aspects of experiments with students are complex and the wisdom of attempting many experiments in man may be questioned. The examples chosen here, however, have been in use for many years and can confidently be regarded as safe.

The first chapter describes procedures such as anaesthesia and dissection, which are common to many of the preparations. After this, the book is divided into sections according to the effects studied; actions affecting the peripheral nervous system, actions affecting the central nervous system, actions on particular organs, and lastly, actions of the body on drugs.

For scientific reasons as well as for legal and moral ones, it is most important to see that laboratory animals are properly cared for. Good experimental results are unlikely to be obtained from animals in poor condition; for example, a sick animal may well die under anaesthesia. The same is true if an animal is frightened.

Any person who works with animals is strongly advised to consult the UFAW handbook, *Care and Management of Laboratory Animals*, 1967, Edinburgh: Livingstone. This gives detailed information about how animals should be housed and fed. It also includes a most useful account of how to handle animals, which should be read to supplement the brief account given below.

Handling Animals

In this book only five species are used, cats, rabbits, guinea-pigs, rats and mice. Wherever possible these should be handled frequently in the animal house. This applies especially to cats and, to a lesser extent, to rats. If a cat is used to being handled and is held by someone with whom it is familiar, it is possible to induce anaesthesia by injection of a barbiturate, or inhalation of halothane without causing any distress. The combination of a frightened animal and a frightened scientist may well cause the animal to die under the anaesthetic, particularly if it is potent.

For anaesthesia with a mask, cats are best held by two people. One grips the scruff of the neck firmly with one hand and the front legs with the other. The second person holds the back legs with one hand and the mask with the other (Fig. 1). If the animal is not frightened, it should not be necessary to put a cloth round the legs to prevent it scratching. A third person may be necessary if the mask is being sprayed with ethyl chloride. It is important that the animal holders should be experienced enough to restrain the animal firmly and not let go, without at the same time gripping it so strongly that they cause pain. Cats suffer extreme distress if they are placed in a box into which ether is blown and even with other volatile anaesthetics the use of a box makes it difficult to gauge the depth of anaesthesia.

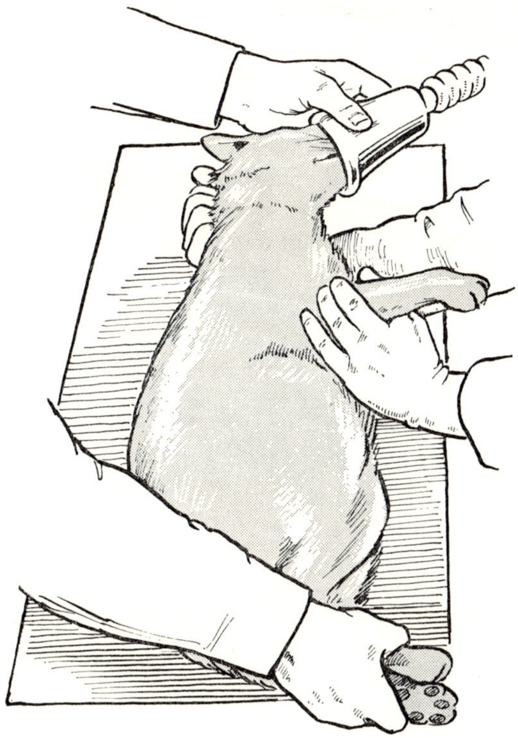

FIG. 1. Holding a cat for anaesthesia.

Rabbits can be held like cats for anaesthesia with a mask. For injections, also, two people are needed, one of whom holds the animal into his side while restraining the front legs, while the second person makes the injection into the marginal vein of the ear (Fig. 2). Rabbits will struggle if placed on a slippery surface but will remain quiet if their feet are on a rough surface and their back is hard up against something. If the rabbit is placed in a box which restrains movement without undue pressure then only one person is needed to make the injection.

Cats and rabbits can be lifted by the scruff of the neck and supported by a hand or arm below. It may be wise to wear gloves but this should be unnecessary if the animals are really tame, in which case it may be easier to lift them with two hands, rather than to use one hand for holding the scruff of the neck. With guinea-pigs, which are much lighter, one hand is usually adequate for lifting them. They appear particularly to like to nestle into corners and can be conveniently carried in the crook of an arm or in the pocket of a laboratory coat. Rats and mice may be lifted by their tails without alarming them though they should be put on a flat surface as soon as possible. If this allows their feet any grip, they will then pull away from where they are held and the scruff of the neck can then be grasped in the other hand. They can thus be held securely while injections are made. Mice can even be held single-handed with the forefinger and thumb holding the scruff of the neck and the little finger holding the tail or legs; the other hand is then free to make an injection (Fig. 3).

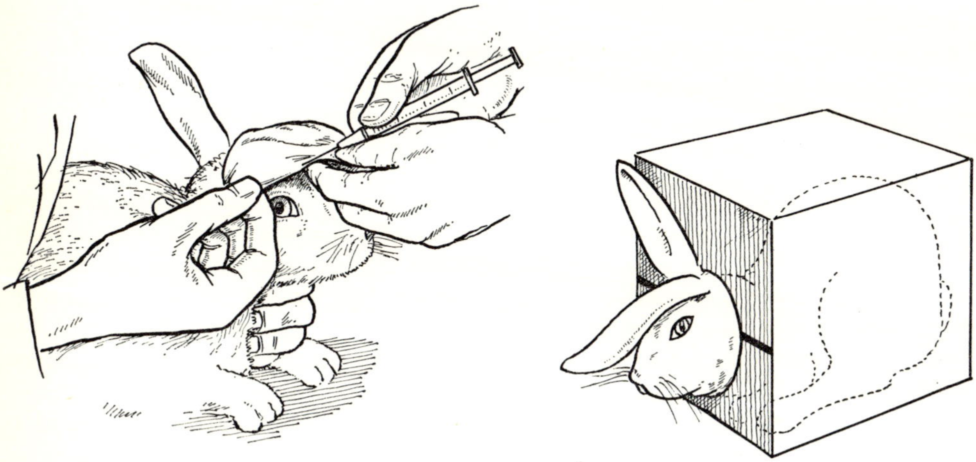

a. b.

FIG. 2. Holding a rabbit; *a*, with an assistant; *b*, rabbit held in a box.

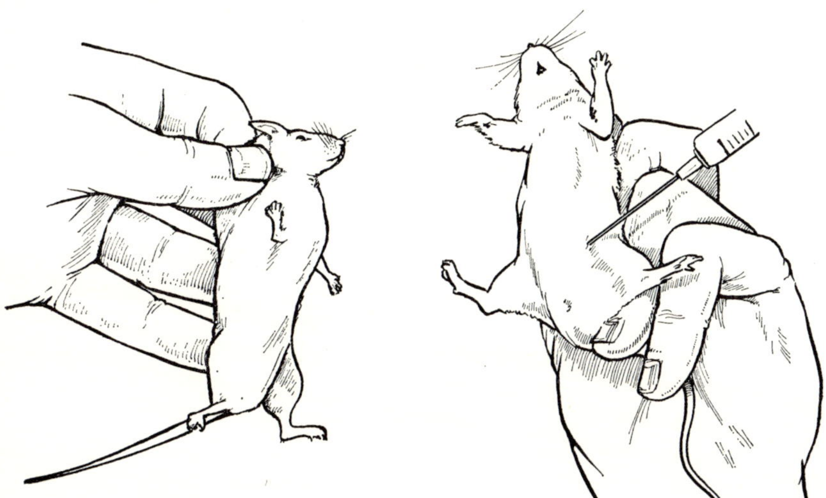

a. b.

FIG. 3. Holding mice; *a*, for lifting; *b*, for an intraperitoneal injection.

Instruments

The choice of instruments depends very much on personal taste but the following instruments are likely to be needed and most of them are illustrated in Figure 4.

Large scissors are needed for general coarse surgery, e.g. for cutting the skin of cats and rabbits and for cutting lint and string. Blunt-ended scissors are convenient for blunt dissection: operating Mayo scissors with a $7\frac{1}{2}$ inch straight conical blade are suitable.

Medium-sized scissors with either straight or curved blades are useful for cutting the skin and soft tissues of small animals and for cutting coarser sutures (1/0 and 3/0). Blunt-ended scissors are convenient for blunt dissection. 5 inch Mayo scissors, straight and curved or flat are suitable.

Medium fine scissors with either straight or curved blades are reserved for cutting blood vessels in cats and rabbits and fine sutures (5/0). Kilner's $4\frac{3}{4}$ inch straight scissors with an extra fine point, and Kilner's $4\frac{3}{4}$ inch curved or flat scissors are suitable.

Fine scissors should only be used for cutting fine blood vessels, e.g. the rat carotid artery and femoral artery or the cat lingual and dorsalis pedis arteries. The Iris, spring action, Birmingham pattern scissors are recommended. Some fine scissors have the blades set at an angle to the handles; this allows the points to be kept up, which is an advantage when cutting connective tissue around vessels, and for cutting fine blood vessels or the dura mater. Brudenall Carter's spring action capsular scissors are suitable.

Large forceps are needed for general work: 6 inch broad, fluted dissecting forceps are suitable. Some people find *large toothed forceps* are convenient for ensuring a firm grip of skin or large masses of tissue but they may tear. Treves dissecting forceps, 6 inch, 2×3 teeth are suitable.

Medium-sized curved forceps are convenient for blunt dissection or for passing ligatures under the trachea or large blood vessels of cats or rabbits. Dental packing forceps with curved points are suitable.

Medium-sized fine toothed forceps are ideal for ensuring a firm grip of smaller pieces of connective tissue or muscle and for holding the cut end of the trachea open. Iris forceps, straight fluted grip, fine tooth 1:2 are suitable.

Medium-sized fine curved forceps are used for delicate blunt dissection, e.g. beneath the trachea of the rat or around blood vessels in most animals, and for passing ligatures. Iris forceps, fluted grip, fully curved, are suitable.

Medium-sized fine straight forceps are needed for delicate blunt dissection. $3\frac{1}{2}$ inch Ophthalmic dissecting forceps are suitable.

Fine pointed forceps are needed for picking up fine sutures, holding open or dilating cut blood vessels, and for stripping connective tissue from small blood vessels and nerves. Watchmakers forceps, 'Dumont' No. 4, are suitable.

Large haemostatic forceps, with straight or curved points, are required for clamping large blood vessels in the cat, or tissue masses containing bleeding vessels. 6 inch Spencer-Wells artery forceps, with either straight or curved points, are suitable. They should have box joints to ensure a firm grip.

Medium-sized haemostatic forceps, with straight or curved points, are useful for clamping small blood vessels in the cat or small tissue masses in the cat or the rat. 5 inch Halstead's 'Mosquito' straight and curved artery forceps are suitable.

Both large and medium artery forceps have ratchets so the pressure between the ends can be adjusted.

Small haemostatic forceps, with straight or curved points (*'Bulldogs'*) are needed for the temporary occlusion of blood vessels. Dieffenbach's artery forceps (straight or curved) are suitable. The 3 cm. size is used for cats and rabbits, the 2 cm. size for rats.

Needle-holding forceps are required for ensuring a firm grip on curved suture needles. Mathieu's spring catch, screw joint, 8 inch forceps are suitable: Spencer-Wells are not.

A fine blunt seeker is very useful for holding open cut blood vessels to aid the insertion of a cannula.

A large scalpel is useful for cutting skin quickly and cleanly. The Swann Morton No. 4 handle is suitable, used with a No. 20 disposable blade.

A medium-sized scalpel is useful for cutting small areas of skin and cutting open the trachea. The Swann Morton No. 3 handle is suitable used with disposable blades Nos. 10 and 11.

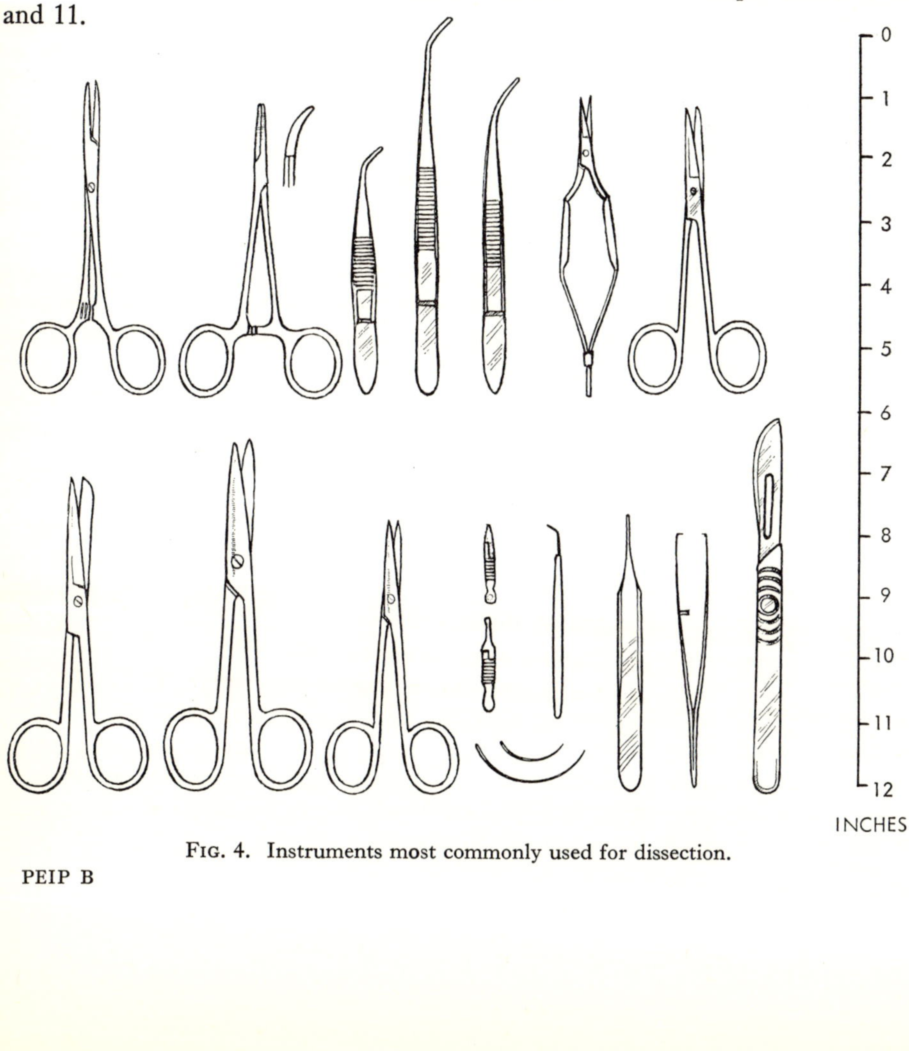

FIG. 4. Instruments most commonly used for dissection.

Cutting needles are necessary for stitching a skin. The smaller No. 3 needles are used for fine work in small animals. Hagedorn, $\frac{1}{2}$ circle needle size, Nos. 3 and 10, and Hagedorn, straight needle size, Nos. 3 and 10, are suitable. Proper *suture* materials are needed for tying off blood vessels. Braided silk sutures of various colours are available on reels. 1/0 is coarse and 5/0 is very fine. Sizes 1/0, 4/0 and 5/0 are particularly useful.

A bone scraper is useful for cleaning the outer surface of bone. Faraboeuf's bone rougine, straight, $6\frac{1}{2}$ inch is suitable.

Dissection

Most of the experiments in this book last for hours only and not for days and the animal is killed at the finish. Aseptic techniques and sophisticated surgery are not required but it is still a good principle to avoid unnecessary exposure of deep tissue or damage to it since this will cause the preparation to deteriorate.

Opening the skin. After clipping or shaving the hair from an area, the skin is either cut open with a sharp scalpel or a longitudinal wedge of skin is cut away with medium or large scissors. The edges are now retracted to expose the underlying tissues and bleeding vessels are cauterized or temporarily clamped with haemostatic forceps. Surgical diathermy may be used instead of a scalpel or scissors for cutting the skin. It is less likely to cause bleeding and may well be essential if large amounts of anticoagulants are to be used.

Blunt dissection is used as much as possible. This involves tearing or pushing through connective tissue along the lines of cleavage. Blunt dissection is either done with the fingers, in large animals, or by inserting closed blunt-ended scissors or forceps and opening them. This method is quick and has the advantage that very small blood vessels seal more easily when their ends are torn than when they are cut. Larger or medium-sized blood vessels should be tied and cut or cauterized and cut to prevent troublesome bleeding later in the experiment, particularly if the blood pressure is made to rise or when an anticoagulant has been given to the animal.

Bleeding. During dissection it sometimes happens that a fairly large blood vessel is accidentally torn or cut and there is a sudden flow of blood. This should be stopped immediately by applying pressure with a swab and finger and thumb. If this is not enough the vessel is identified, clamped off with haemostatic forceps and tied. To tie off a vessel that is already cut, check that the thread is placed between the cut end of the vessel, secured by the clamp and the tissue. It is often convenient to pass the tie loosely round the clamp, pull it down to the tip and slide it off onto the vessel. It is always better, however, to anticipate trouble and to tie off even quite small vessels before cutting or tearing them. To tie off a vessel before cutting it, two threads (5/0 for small vessels, 3/0 for larger ones) are passed under it and then tied at least 2 mm. apart. The ends of these threads are held taut so that the vessel is slightly stretched. The vessel is cut and the ends of the threads then trimmed. If an electric cautery or diathermy is available it is convenient to coagulate small vessels instead of tying them and this saves considerable time. There are two main types of cautery tip, one of which can be used for cutting and the other, which is very small, for sealing small vessels.

Injections

For any injection the needle must be sharp and of suitable size (Table I). Even if

TABLE I

		I.V.	I.P.	S.C.	I.M.	Oral
Mouse	Needle size	27 G $\frac{1}{2}$ in.	25 G $\frac{3}{4}$ in.	25 G $\frac{3}{4}$ in.	25 G $\frac{3}{4}$ in.	18 G 2 in.
	Max. dose volume	0·4 ml.	1ml.	0·4 ml	0·4 ml.	1 ml.
Rat	Needle size	—	25 G 1 in.	25 G 1 in.	25 G 1 in.	—
	Max. dose volume	—	2 ml.	1 ml.	0·4 ml.	—
Cat	Needle size	—	21 G $1\frac{1}{2}$ in.	25 G 1 in.	25 G 1 in.	—
	Max. dose volume	—	5 ml.	2 ml.	2 ml.	—
Rabbit	Needle size	25 G 1 in.	21 G $1\frac{1}{2}$ in.	25 G 1 in.	25 G 1 in.	no. 9 catheter
	Max. dose volume	10 ml.	5 ml.	2 ml.	2 ml.	5–10 ml.
Guinea-pig	Needle size	—	25 G 1 in.	25 G 1 in.	25 G 1 in.	—
	Max. dose volume	—	2–4 ml.	1 ml.	0·5 ml.	—

it need not be sterile, there is no justification for re-using it if it is at all blunt, because disposable needles are not expensive. Disposable syringes, too, are cheap and much more robust than glass ones. Though it is just possible that some drugs may dissolve slightly in the plastic, this does not usually necessitate using glass ones. In many experiments sterility does not matter, and syringes, as opposed to needles, may be re-used many times, especially if they are being used always for the same drug solution. In these circumstances an appreciable saving in expense is made by re-using 'disposable' plastic syringes. These can even be used for different drugs provided they are well washed. A few drugs are reputedly particularly difficult to wash out and it is probably wisest to use a fresh syringe, for example, with secondary or tertiary bases, but with quaternary salts the useful life of a syringe can be very long, being limited only by the tendency for the graduation to become worn away. This can be reduced by placing transparent tape over

the markings. The main disadvantage of using plastic syringes is the difficulty of dislodging air bubbles trapped on the sides. It may be necessary to tap the syringe quite sharply several times to remove them. Some syringes are so designed that small bubbles are not likely to enter the needle but it is always important to check that no air is injected. At present all plastic syringes have Luer fittings and this pattern is becoming standard. It may be difficult to obtain very fine needles, e.g. for the injection into the tail of the mouse, for which a 27 gauge needle is required, with Luer fittings. Needles with Record fittings and glass Record syringes will then be required.

The most frequently used methods of injection are subcutaneous, intraperitoneal, intramuscular, intravenous and oral. For a subcutaneous injection the skin is lifted up and the needle pushed firmly through it. The point of the needle should be quite free to move between the skin and the muscle. If the needle is of a suitable length or the syringe is held with the hand below it (Fig. 5) there is no possibility of inserting the needle too far into the animal. The position of the hand can then be altered so that the thumb presses the plunger. Either side of the back of an animal is most suitable for a subcutaneous injection. If there is no one available to hold the animal, however, it may be necessary to make the injection higher up towards the head because one hand will be needed to hold the scruff of the neck of the animal. In this way it is possible for one person to inject mice, rats or guinea-pigs and it is sometimes possible to inject docile rabbits or cats without assistance.

For an intraperitoneal injection the procedure is similar to that for a subcutaneous one, but it is the skin of the abdomen which must be held taut. The animal should be gripped by the scruff of the neck and by its tail or hind limbs, though with rats it may be better to place the hand right round the shoulders and hold the forelegs crossed firmly over the chest (Fig. 6). With rabbits it is advisable to hold the animal close against one's body (Fig. 7). The needle is pushed firmly through the abdomen in a region where it is not likely to penetrate the liver, kidney, spleen or bladder and the plunger pressed.

For an intramuscular injection the procedure is similar to the subcutaneous injection except that the site must be a muscular part of the body, usually in the region of the thigh or buttock. With this injection the tip of the needle should not be free but should have penetrated the muscle.

For an intravenous injection the procedure varies from one species to another. In the experiments in this book, intravenous injections in cats, guinea-pigs and rats are made under anaesthesia. In conscious rabbits, however, injections can be made into the marginal vein of the ear. The rabbit is held suitably (p. 4) and the fur is removed from the vein at the top outside edge of the ear either by plucking or with clippers. The vein is made to distend by occluding the flow at the base of the ear with the thumb and forefinger. It is advisable to shine a lamp on the ear (not directly on the face of the rabbit). This serves to warm the ear as well as to illuminate it. It may also be necessary to rub the edge of the ear gently. A needle can easily be inserted into the vein when it is distended, the thumb and forefinger released and the plunger of the syringe pressed in (Fig. 8). As a general principle the plunger of the syringe should be withdrawn to see if blood appears, though this should not be done with the mouse tail vein injection.

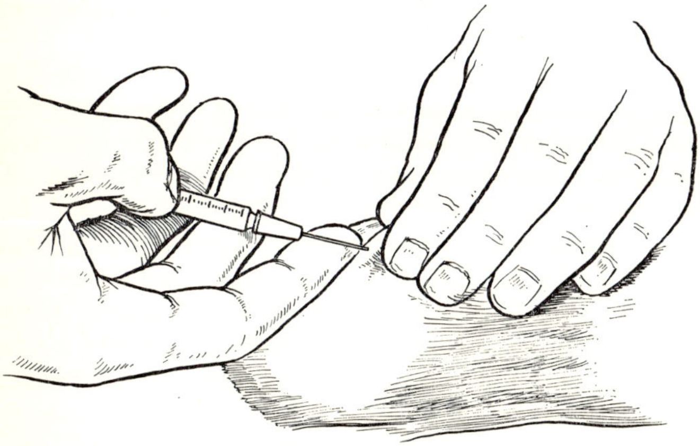

FIG. 5. A subcutaneous injection. The skin is lifted up and the needle inserted at an angle of about 45°.

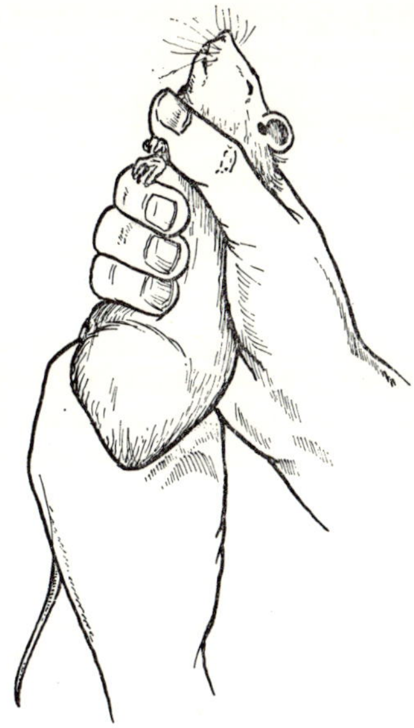

FIG. 6. Holding a rat.

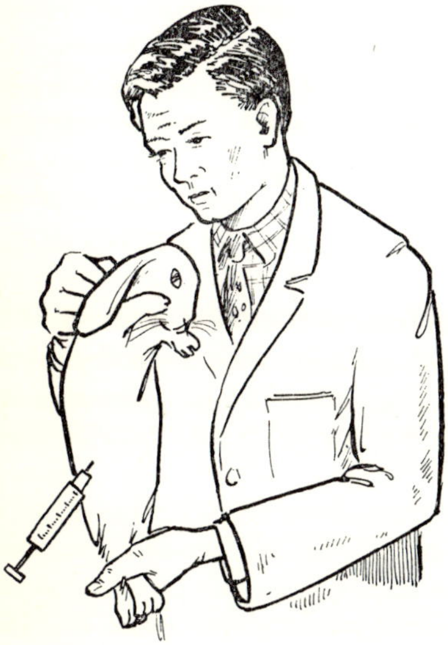

FIG. 7. Holding a rabbit for an intraperitoneal injection.

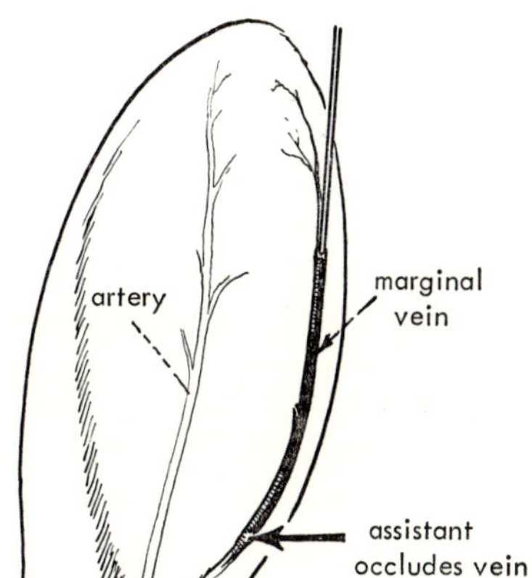

FIG. 8. Injection into marginal vein of rabbit's ear.

If the needle is not correctly placed it is best to remove it and to repeat the attempt. It is always wisest to start as far away from the base of the ear as possible to allow a number of attempts to be made. To avoid the needle being dislodged from the vein if the animal moves its head, it is often convenient to attach the needle to the syringe by way of a length of plastic tubing (e.g. a scalp-vein needle set). The needle can then be held in place with a piece of adhesive tape and the injection made at a distance from the animal.

In mice, intravenous injections are made into the tail vein. The animal is placed in a tube which is stoppered so that its tail protrudes (Fig. 9). The vein is made to dilate by placing the tail in warm water (45 to 50° C).The tip of the tail is held with the finger and thumb of one hand and the injection made with the syringe held in the other hand. There are four tail veins in the mouse, any of which will do. As with the injection into the rabbit ear vein, it is advisable to start as far away from the base as possible, to allow for more than one attempt. If the needle is not in the vein the injection will produce a white area around the tip of the needle; if it is in place, the plunger can be pressed with little effort. With this injection there is a tendency for the blood to clot in the fine needle and it is best not to try to withdraw blood to see if the needle is correctly placed. This technique requires practice and should only be attempted with albino mice in which the tail vein can easily be seen. It is advisable to use a very fine needle (27 gauge, $\frac{1}{2}$ inch).

For an oral injection a suitable stomach tube is necessary. With mice a No. 2 serum needle is used, which has no point or bevel. Similar needles can be made by filing off the point of a 2 inch × 18 gauge injection needle. The animal is held with one hand by the scruff of the neck (as for an intraperitoneal injection, p. 5) with the mouth held so that the oesophagus is as straight as possible. The tube is then carefully inserted between the tongue and the roof of the mouth (Fig. 10). Once past the larynx the tube should move easily and it may be necessary to mark the needle to indicate how far it should be inserted (usually this is between 30 mm and 40 mm). This technique, like the injection into the tail vein, requires practice. Faulty injections (e.g. into the lungs) usually cause immediate death.

With rabbits a No. 9 rubber catheter is used, inserted through a hole in a wooden or plastic gag placed behind the front teeth. The technique requires considerable practice and it is often best to administer a short-lasting anaesthetic such as intravenous thiopentone sodium (up to 20 mg./kg.), so that the tube can be passed easily. The catheter is covered with glycerol or some other surgical lubricant and connected to a funnel into which the drug solution is poured.

The suggested limits to the volumes which may be administered by a particular route are shown in Table I.

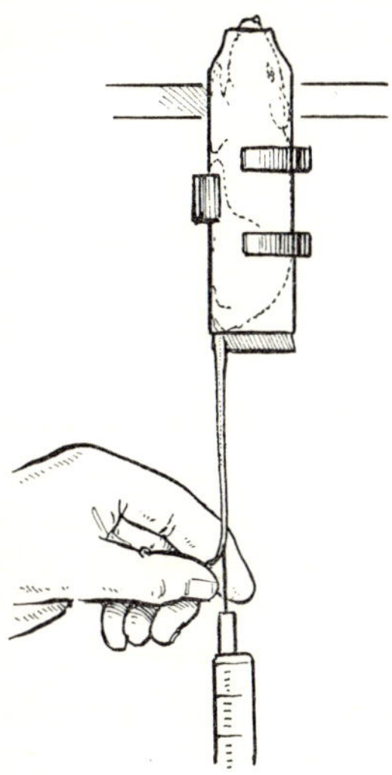

FIG. 9. Intravenous injection in a mouse.

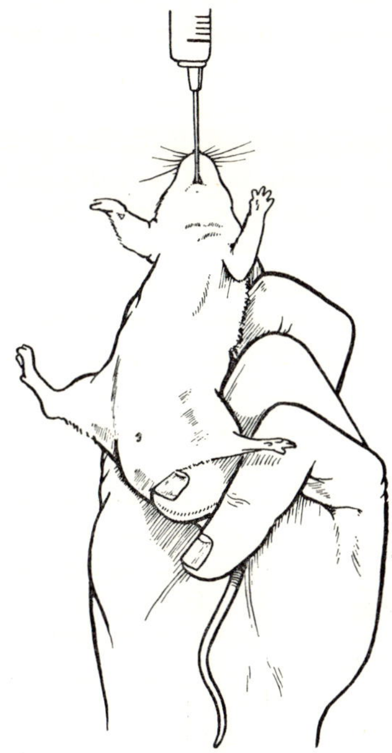

FIG. 10. Oral injection in a mouse.

Cannulation

Successful cannulation depends upon having cannulae of the right size and shape (Fig. 11). For insertion into the trachea, glass cannulae are particularly suitable because they are transparent and also because they can easily be cleaned. For arteries and veins much finer cannulae are needed and it is easier to make these out of plastic than out of glass. Polyethylene or nylon tubing is drawn out in a very small flame. The technique used is similar to that for glass except that these plastics soften at much lower temperatures. The two materials behave differently and nylon is easier to work. After practice, cannulae can be made with tips as small as 0·25 mm. The nylon cannulae are stiffer than the others and consequently less likely to collapse when the vessel is tied onto them.

Fine plastic tubing is particularly useful because it makes it possible to place the injection block at a convenient distance from the site of the injection, so that there is no risk of dislodging the cannula. The dead space is extremely small, even with several centimetres of, for example, 0·9 mm. internal diameter tubing. This can be inserted directly into the femoral or cephalic vein of a cat, though it must be pulled down to about 0·25 to 0·5 mm. at the tip before it can be inserted into the femoral vein of the rat.

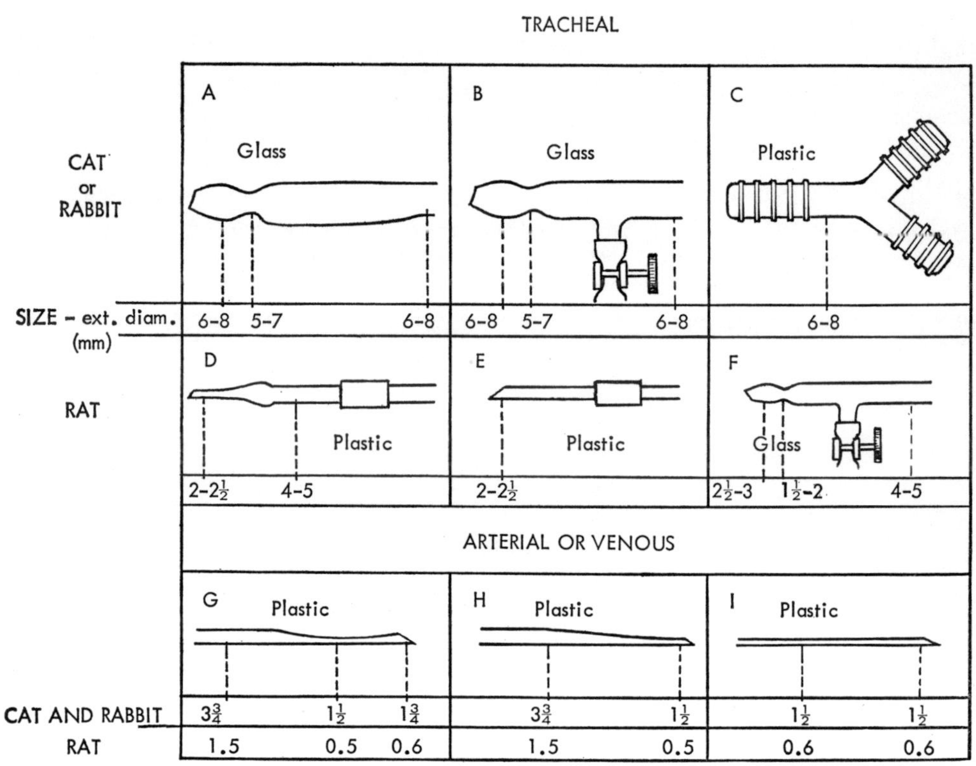

FIG. 11. Details of cannulae.

An injection block made of araldite or other plastic makes a convenient means of injecting a drug and washing it in, but if a minimum amount of dead space is required, the other apparatus shown in Figure 12 is recommended.

As with injections from a syringe, it is most important to ensure that no air is injected at any time. To prevent clots forming in these fine tubes it is important to fill them with 0·9 per cent sodium chloride containing heparin, 50 units/ml., before inserting them.

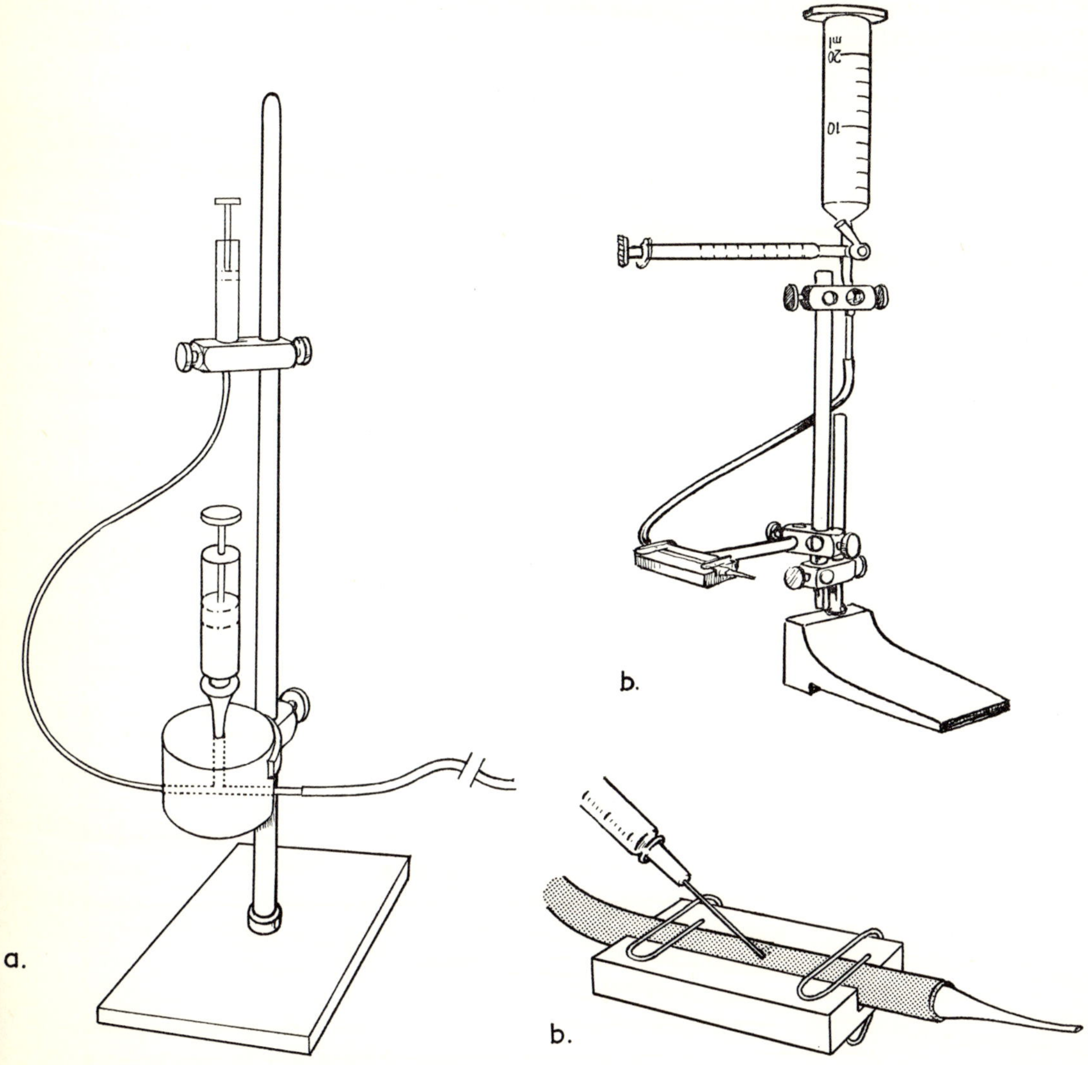

FIG. 12. Apparatus for repeated intravenous injections; *a*, T-junction set in plastic; *b*, 3-way tap or alternatively (inset) injection made through rubber tubing attached to cannula. Injections are made from the small syringe and washed in with saline from the large syringe.

1. *Cannulation of the trachea* (cat, rabbit and rat, Fig. 13). When anaesthesia has been induced and the animal is unconscious and flaccid (p. 18), the front of the neck is shaved with electric clippers or the fur cut off with scissors (this can be omitted with the rat). The larynx is felt as a lump through the skin, and below it a length of skin is picked up and cut open with scissors or a scalpel. This exposes the longitudinal muscles in front of the trachea. Blunt dissection along the midline is used to divide these. The trachea can now be seen and is freed from connective tissue with curved iris forceps or dental packing forceps depending on the species. Two strong ligatures are passed around the trachea but not tied. A cut is made in the trachea between the two ligatures big enough to allow the insertion of the cannula. The top ligature is tied and pulled towards the head. This makes it easy to push the cannula in. It may be necessary to hold the cut end of the trachea open with forceps while this is being done. The second ligature is now tied around the cannula, the free ends of the ligature furthest from the lungs are also tied loosely round the cannula to keep it properly aligned.

2. *Cannulation of a vein* (cat, rabbit and rat, Fig. 14). The choice of vein depends upon its size and the convenience of its position. Mostly the femoral vein is selected. The external jugular vein is sometimes used but it has many branches which must be tied off. In cats the cephalic vein is a suitable alternative to the femoral vein. When the vein has been located a length of about 10 mm. must be prepared free from connective tissue and any branches are tied off. Mostly this is done by blunt dissection with curved forceps but fine pointed forceps may be needed to ensure that all the connective tissue sheath around the vein has been stripped away. This avoids the possibility that the cannula will be inserted between the vein and the connective tissue instead of into the vein. If the veins collapse or go into a spasm while they are being stripped (which frequently occurs with the rat or the rabbit), they should be swabbed with warm saline and made to distend (see below).

When a suitable length of vein has been prepared, the blood flow is occluded by placing a bulldog clip on the end nearest to the heart. Two threads (5/0 for a rat, 3/0 for a rabbit or cat) are carefully passed around the vein and half-tied, i.e. the threads are crossed over but not pulled tight. The vein is then made to distend fully by using a finger to push blood towards the bulldog clip. The thread furthest from the heart is now tied firmly and held taut so as to stretch the vein slightly. This thread is held by an assistant or by a 'third hand' (an adjustable holder) or can be clipped to the skin with a pair of haemostatic forceps. A small cut is made, not more than halfway through the vein, as near to the tied thread as possible, i.e. as far from the bulldog clip as possible so that, if the cannulation is unsuccessful there is room for a further attempt. The cut should be made at an angle (Fig. 14) so that there is a small flap which can be lifted up with a fine seeker or held with a fine pair of forceps while the cannula is inserted. If desired the bulldog clip can be removed so that the cannula can be pushed further in still. The second thread is now tied around this cannula and the bulldog removed, if this has not been done already. The first thread is now tied around the cannula to keep it aligned correctly. The cannula and the tubing connected to it should have been filled with saline containing heparin (50 units/ml.) before any attempt is made to insert it.

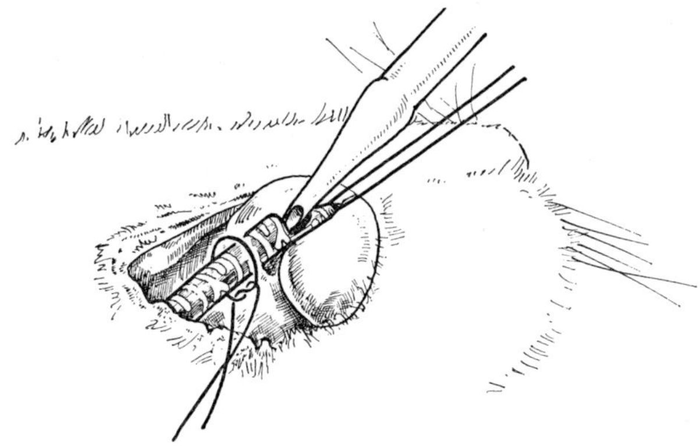

FIG. 13. Insertion of a tracheal cannula.

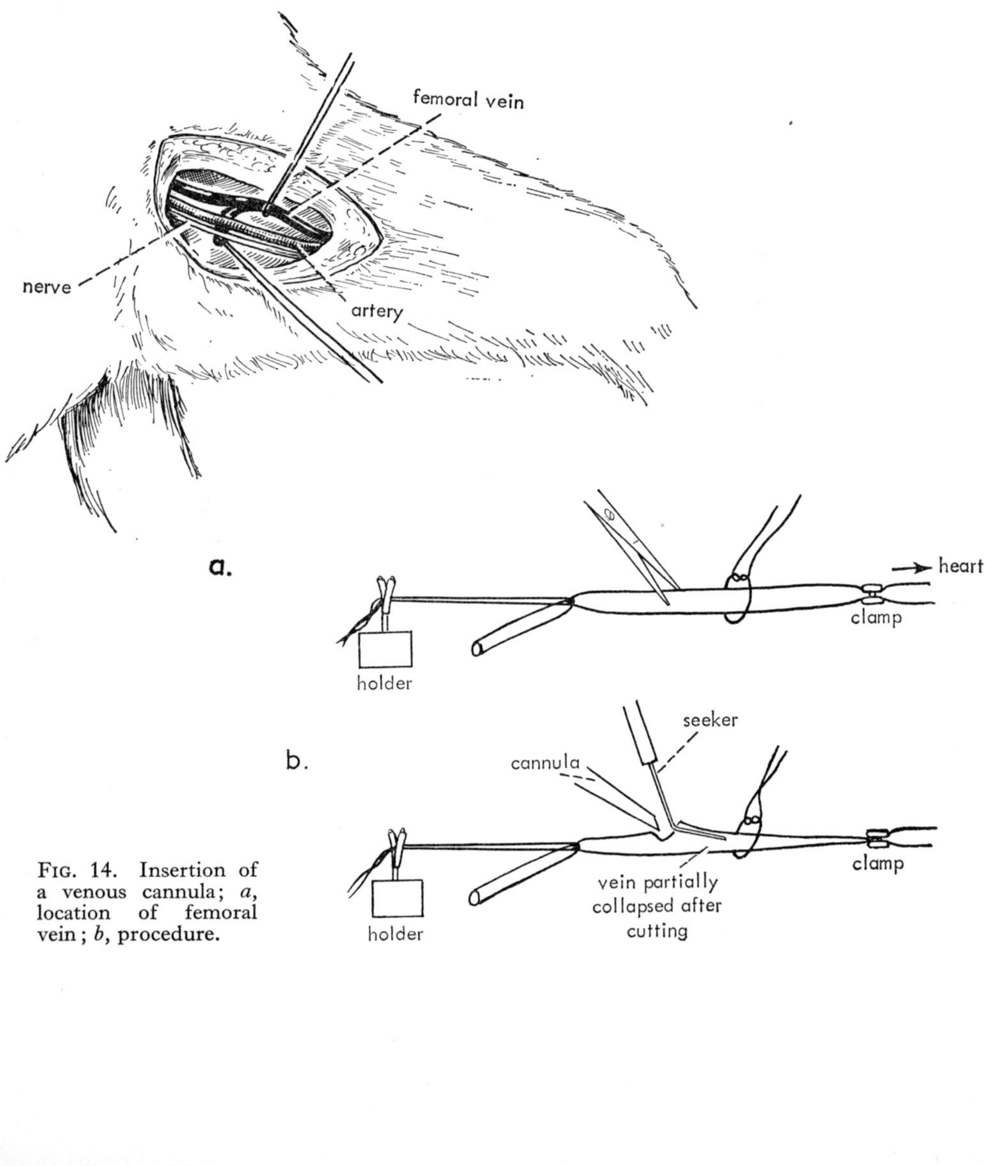

FIG. 14. Insertion of a venous cannula; *a*, location of femoral vein; *b*, procedure.

3. *Cannulation of an artery* (cat, rabbit, rat). The usual reason for cannulating an artery is to record the blood pressure and for this the carotid artery is most convenient. In the cat's superior cervical ganglion preparation, however, the blood pressure is often recorded from the femoral artery. The procedure for inserting the cannula is very similar to the cannulation of a vein. Two ligatures are passed round the cleaned length of artery. The thread furthest from the heart is now tied and then, when the artery is distended with blood, the bulldog clip is placed at the end nearest to the heart. The arterial cannula (Fig. 11) is now prepared. It should be connected to a mercury manometer or to the blood pressure transducer through a three-way tap with a syringe full of heparinized saline attached (Fig. 15). The connection between the three-way tap and the transducer or manometer is closed and all the air bubbles in the arterial cannula flushed out with heparinized saline and the tap set so as to close off the arterial cannula. A slanting cut is made in the artery between the tied ligature and the bulldog clip. The cannula is inserted and tied into place. The pressure in the manometer or transducer is raised, by means of the syringe, to the expected blood pressure of the animal. The tap is set so that the syringe is closed off and the arterial cannula is connected to the recording device. If there are no leaks in the system the pressure will remain steady. The bulldog clip can now be removed. If the arterial pressure has been correctly guessed there will be little flow of blood out of the animal into the cannula. As an added precaution to prevent clotting, the animal is given heparin (1,000 units/kg. i.v.).

The need for heparin to prevent clots forming is greater with arterial cannulae than with venous cannulae. This is because a clot in a venous cannula can easily be dislodged by pressure but the direction of the flow forces any clot back into an arterial cannula. It is, nevertheless, worth trying to dislodge a clot in an arterial cannula, using the syringe and three-way tap (Fig. 15).

In the experiments with the cat tibialis muscle and superior cervical ganglion preparations (pp. 37 and 49) drugs are injected intra-arterially. The procedure is exactly the same as in the cannulation of an artery for recording the blood pressure, but it is most important that the three-way tap should not leak and that it be kept closed except when injections are being made. The injection is made against the arterial pressure, which is quite enough to displace the plunger of a syringe, so it is important to make sure that there is no chance of the blood forcing its way into the injection system at any time.

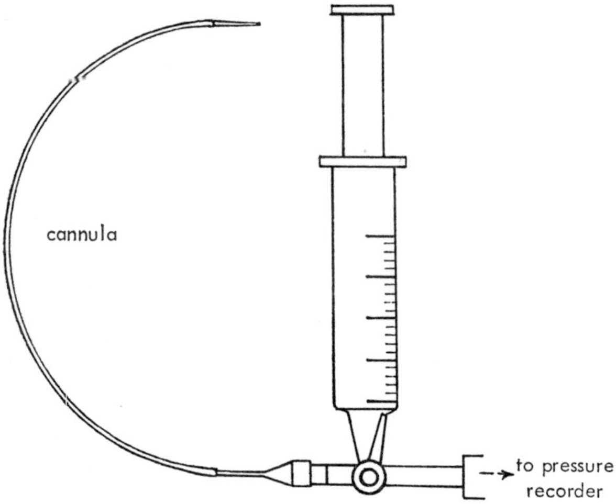

FIG. 15. Attachment for recording arterial blood-pressure. The large syringe attached to the 3-way tap contains heparinized saline.

Anaesthesia

Cats. Before attempting to anaesthetize an animal, a suitable respiration pump or a cyclator (Fig. 16) must be available, together with all the connections necessary for connecting it to the particular size of animal and to the anaesthetic machine. Whenever respiration is inadequate it should be assisted even though the animal may still be breathing spontaneously. The anaesthetic vapours will have to be introduced into the inflow of the pump. If the animal has actually stopped breathing it will not be exhaling the anaesthetic vapour and the first priority is to re-establish ventilation.

Anaesthesia may be induced by the inhalation of agents such as halothane, ether, trichlorethylene, methoxyflurane, cyclopropane and ethylchloride. The highest concentrations of nitrous oxide which can be given (80 per cent plus 20 per cent oxygen) are not potent enough to induce anaesthesia in cats but are frequently used in conjunction with halothane in order to reduce the amounts of this expensive agent which need to be used. In most circumstances, however, it is usual to maintain anaesthesia in cats by administering another agent intravenously, e.g. chloralose, urethane or a barbiturate. Alternatively, anaesthesia can be both induced and maintained by the intraperitoneal injection of urethane or barbiturate.

Halothane, 3 to 4 per cent, is the most suitable agent for induction. It is given from an anaesthetic machine, with a calibrated halothane dispenser, either along with pure oxygen or with a mixture of nitrous oxide (75 to 80 per cent) and oxygen. As soon as the animal is relaxed it is tied to the operating table and the level of halothane in the inspired gas reduced to 1 per cent. This is important because halothane is potent and the high concentration used for induction will be fatal if continued.

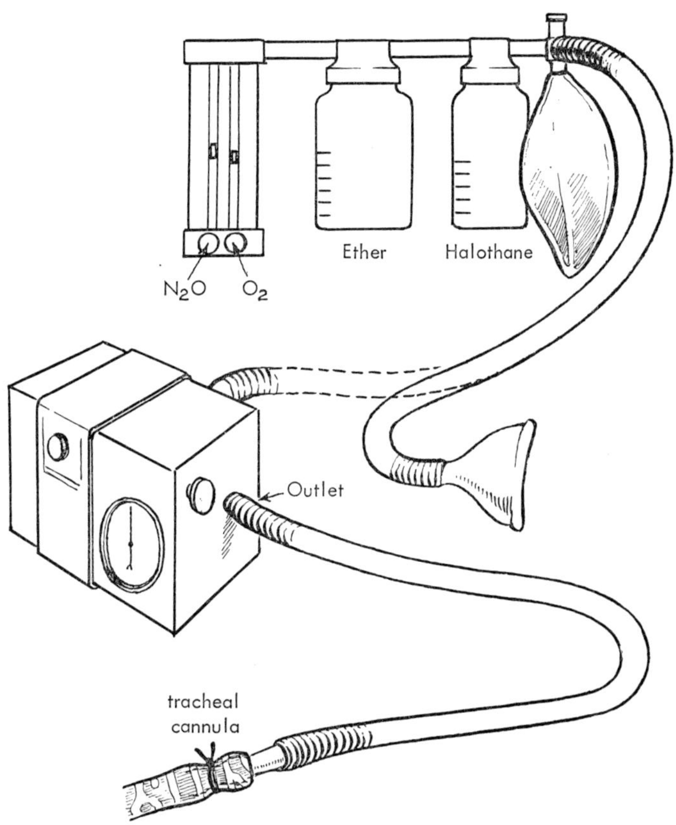

FIG. 16. Cyclator. After induction of anaesthesia with a mask, a tracheal cannula is inserted, which is attached to the Cyclator, which replaces the mask (as indicated by the dotted lines).

A popular but unsatisfactory alternative for inducing anaesthesia is to spray ethyl-chloride into a conical mask containing a plug of absorbent cotton wool at its apex. As with any volatile anaesthetic, it is advisable to hold the mask near the animal and allow it to inhale the fumes for a minute or two before placing the mask firmly on the animal. As soon as the animal is anaesthetised the ethyl chloride is replaced by ether. Induction with ethyl chloride is rapid and the anaesthetic dose is hard to gauge. Accidental overdose and cardiac arrest, probably due to sensitization of the myocardium to adrenaline, are much more prone to occur than with halothane. Ether alone should not be used for induction because it is distressing to the animal and the experimenter, is very slow and causes excessive salivary and bronchial secretions.

Once anaesthesia has been induced it is advisable to insert the tracheal cannula before attempting to insert a venous cannula. The tracheal cannula makes it easy to administer inhalation anaesthetics and allows rapid and simple artificial ventilation by a pump in the case of accidental respiratory arrest, which is very liable to occur when an intravenous anaesthetic is given to an animal following induction with a volatile anaesthetic. When the trachea has been cut the animal is no longer inhaling anaesthetic but there should be no danger of its regaining consciousness. Normally the insertion of the tracheal cannula only takes a few seconds and if there is any delay, anaesthetic vapour can easily be applied directly to the hole in the trachea. When the tracheal cannula has been inserted, it is rapidly connected to the anaesthetic machine, used as an open circuit with $\frac{1}{2}$ to 1 per cent halothane and a flow rate of 2 litres/min., or to a Woulfe's bottle containing ether through which oxygen or air is steadily blown.

The femoral or cephalic veins are now cannulated as described on page 16. Whatever the nature of the intravenous anaesthetic to be administered, it is absolutely essential to give it very slowly to avoid the risk of complete respiratory and circulatory collapse. It is advisable to stop administering the volatile anaesthetic and to wait for some signs of lightening consciousness, such as increased respiration, increased muscle tone or tendency to spontaneous movement, or reappearance of the corneal reflex, before giving the intravenous anaesthetic.

For cats the maintenance anaesthetic frequently used is chloralose, 40 to 80 mg./kg.; this produces deep anaesthesia lasting for about 6 hours; muscle tone is high and the animals react vigorously to loud noises. Pentobarbitone sodium, 30 to 40 mg./kg., produces anaesthesia lasting for only 2 to 3 hours, and a further dose will be needed subsequently. A mixture of diallylbarbituric acid and urethane (Dial Compound), 0·35 ml./kg. given intraperitoneally is very popular both for induction and maintenance of anaesthesia. Barbiturates are not very satisfactory for experiments on ganglia because they themselves depress ganglionic transmission.

In experiments where it is important to keep the depth of anaesthesia controlled within narrow limits, it is better to maintain the level with an intravenous infusion rather than by giving repeated injections.

Rabbits and rats. Usually in these species the same anaesthetic is used for induction and for maintenance and is given by injection. In experiments in which the animal recovers, however, it may be more convenient and safer to use a volatile anaesthetic, such as halothane, and techniques for doing this with small animals have been described by Parbrook (1966)[1].

For rabbits and rats urethane is frequently used and with rabbits a mixture of chloralose and urethane ((Table II) is popular. With rabbits the dose is administered gradually into the marginal vein of the ear (p. 11); anaesthesia is achieved well before the full dose has been given and the remainder of the anaesthetic is given slowly over about 15 minutes.

With rats it is convenient to give half the anaesthetic dose by the intraperitoneal route and, when the animal is partly anaesthetized, to give the remainder subcutaneously. It may be necessary to wait 20 to 30 minutes before the rat is fully anaesthetized. This method combines the relatively rapid onset of the intraperitoneal injection with the more prolonged duration of the subcutaneous injection. It has been found that less satisfactory results are obtained when the entire dose is given by one route.

Pentobarbitone sodium (30 to 40 mg. i.p.) is quite a satisfactory alternative to urethane in rats for short procedures. The effects of a single anaesthetic dose do not last for as long as urethane, and in addition male rats metabolise barbiturates more rapidly than female rats and so will require even more frequent maintenance doses.

Ventilation. Some preparations (e.g. the pithed rat) must be ventilated artificially. In other experiments (e.g. with neuromuscular blocking agents) artificial respiration may be necessary because the animal's breathing has become inadequate. The rate and volume of respiration are most important and the following are recommended: for cats and rabbits, 20 strokes/min., each of 12 ml./kg. (i.e. 240 ml./kg./min.); for rats 50 strokes/min., each of 8 ml./kg. (i.e. 400 ml./kg./min.).

Temperature maintenance during anaesthesia. During anaesthesia it is usually necessary to warm the animal because its temperature-regulating mechanism is not functioning normally. The operating table itself may be heated, or the animal may be placed on a small electric blanket. Alternatively the animal may be heated by an overhead infra-red lamp. Whatever method is used, it is important to check the rectal temperature of the animal and to see that it is maintained within normal limits; for the cat, $38{\cdot}6° \pm 1{\cdot}0$°C, for the rabbit $38{\cdot}4° \pm 1{\cdot}0$°C, for the rat $37{\cdot}3° \pm 0{\cdot}5$°C. Ideally a feedback circuit is used so that the animal's temperature controls the heat source and when the animal gets too cold the heat is switched on. Suitable commercial equipment is available (see also Krnjević and Mitchell (1961)[2].

[1] Parbrook, G. D. (1966). *Anaesthesia*, **21**, 403–405.
[2] Krnjević, K. & Mitchell, J. F. (1961). *J. Physiol.*, **158**, 6P.

TABLE II

I = induction; M = maintenance

Method	Anaesthetic	Dose	Suitable for	Comments
Anaesthetic machine	Nitrous oxide/oxygen (4:1) with halothane	I = 3 to 4% M = $\frac{1}{2}$ to $\frac{3}{4}$% halothane	Cats and rabbits. Rats can be anaesthetized by blowing the gases into a closed box containing the animal. Induction and recovery are rapid.	If higher concentrations of halothane are used respiration may be depressed. Nitrous oxide will not anaesthetize cats by itself, but it reduces the amount of halothane required to induce anaesthesia. Halothane lowers the blood pressure because it causes vasodilatation, and there may also be troublesome bleeding. Prolonged use can cause cardiac arrythmias.
Open-drop mask	Ether	I = a sufficient quantity	Cats, rats and rabbits	Ether causes excessive bronchial secretion, but it can safely be used if the animal is injected with atropine (1 mg./kg.) before the anaesthesia is induced. Atropine must not be used in the cat superior cervical ganglion preparation (p. 49). Ether will often stop the heart before it stops respiration and the clinical condition of the animal should be watched very closely.
Open-drop mask	Ethyl chloride	I = a sufficient quantity	Cats and rabbits	Induction is very fast and cardiac arrest is likely. Following induction ether should be used for maintenance anaesthesia. Ethyl chloride often stops heart before respiration (see ether).
Intravenous	Thiopentone sodium	I only; up to 20 mg./kg. Not recommended for maintenance	Cats and rabbits	Thiopentone is rather cumulative if used for a prolonged period.

Method	Anaesthetic	Dose	Suitable for	Comments
Intravenous	Pentobarbitone sodium	I and M. 30 to 40 mg./kg.	Cats, rabbits, rats	Moderately long acting.
Intravenous injection	Chloralose	M 40 to 80 mg./kg.	Cats and rabbits	Chloralose is a safe anaesthetic in nearly all instances. It is generally given by intravenous injection, but can also be administered by the intraperitoneal route.
Intravenous injection or intra-peritoneal	Urethane	I and M up to 1·75 g./kg.	Rats and rabbits Sometimes cats	
Intravenous or intra-peritoneal	Urethane and Chloralose	I and M 500 mg./kg. 40 mg./kg.	Rabbits and cats	
Intravenous or intra-peritoneal	'Dial' compound (diallylbarbituric acid and urethane)	I and M 70 mg./kg. 280 mg./kg.		

Correction of acidosis. If an anaesthetic is given for a long time, animals develop acidosis. This should be corrected by administering sodium bicarbonate. Ideally the bicarbonate concentration should be measured at regular intervals, but even if this is not done, it is advisable to infuse sodium bicarbonate (a molar solution is convenient) at the rate of 1 to 1·5 mMol./kg. body weight per hour. In long lasting experiments the likelihood of fluctuations in the plasma concentrations of other ions such as potassium should be considered, particularly if consistent responses of excitable tissues to a drug are required.

Killing Animals

To kill an animal at the end of an experiment, a large intravenous injection of air may be given. Alternatively cats and rabbits may be killed with 1 ml. of a very strong solution of barbiturate (Expiral, 200 mg./ml. pentobarbitone sodium). Smaller doses, e.g. 0·2 ml., are required for rats. Urethane, 250 mg./ml. is also suitable in doses of 7 ml./kg. Mice can be killed very quickly by placing them in a jar containing cotton wool soaked in chloroform.

The Spinal and Decerebrate Animal

If the respiration is maintained, the circulation will continue to function in an animal even though the central nervous system has been destroyed. In these circumstances drugs can produce effects only by actions on the peripheral nervous system and it may be possible to assess how far drugs act centrally, and how far they act peripherally, by comparing their effects before and after destroying the brain. There are legal advantages, too, in working with an animal whose brain has been destroyed, because the animal is technically dead.

In the decerebrate animal the cerebral hemispheres are destroyed but the midbrain and medulla are not. The respiratory centre is therefore intact and the animal should continue to breathe unaided. The thermo-regulating centres should also be intact but they are likely to be damaged if the decerebration is not skilfully performed. In the spinal animal the medulla and the midbrain are destroyed as well as the cerebral hemispheres, the spinal cord being cut in the region between the occipital bone and the first vertebra. The animal must therefore be ventilated artificially and its temperature also carefully controlled.

For preparing either the decerebrate or the spinal animal it is first anaesthetized with a volatile anaesthetic but from then on the procedures are different and are described separately. Details are given in Burn, J. H. *Practical Pharmacology* (1952, Oxford: Blackwell) but the following account includes some modifications.

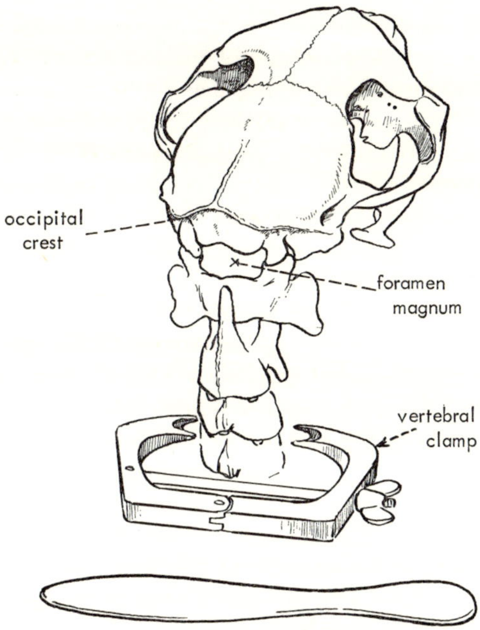

FIG. 17. Cat's skull and spinal column, to illustrate the procedure for preparing a spinal cat, and point of applying a vertebral clamp. The decerebrating probe, shown below, should be about 1 cm. in width, so as to pass easily into a hole 1·5 cm. square (p. 26).

The spinal cat. The anaesthetized animal is placed on its back and both carotid arteries are tied as high as possible in the neck. The animal is then placed on its abdomen and the head is flexed forward on to the neck, care being taken to see that the tracheal cannula and trachea are not kinked. A longitudinal cut is made in the midline from the middle of the skull down to the back of the neck. The skin is retracted and the occipital crest is seen, or can be felt, as a V-shaped ridge at the back of the skull (Fig. 17). The neck muscles are now either separated longitudinally in the midline by blunt dissection for a distance of 3 cm. below the occipital crest, or are divided transversely with a cautery knife below the occipital crest on to the occipital bone. When the muscle layers are retracted, the occipital bone at the back of the skull and the first cervical vertebra are exposed. The cisterna magna can be felt between the two bones as a fluid-filled mass; when this is cleaned it becomes transparent and the underlying spinal cord may be seen. The level of anaesthesia is now deepened to reduce reflex movements when the cord is cut. The animal is connected to the respiratory pump, the cisterna magna is opened and the spinal cord cut with a thick blunt-edged probe about 5 mm. wide by 1 to 2 mm. thick. A special rod, maximum diameter 5 mm., is now pushed up into the brain through the opening at the base of the skull, the foramen magnum, and stirred round in order to destroy the brain.

In addition to tying the carotid arteries the vertebral arteries can be occluded by placing a clamp between the side processes of the second and third cervical vertebrae. This arrests the cerebral circulation completely and thus reduces the loss of blood when the brain is destroyed with the rod. The signs of arrest of the circulation and of death of the brain are fixed dilated pupils, absence of reflexes involving the head and respiratory arrest. If the use of the vertebral artery clamp has killed the brain it is not necessary to destroy it mechanically with the rod, but it may be wisest to do so as an extra precaution.

Decerebrate cat. For this operation a decerebrating probe is needed. This must be blunt-ended and can easily be made from a scalpel handle or spoon handle suitably bent.

After the tracheal cannula has been inserted, the animal is placed on its abdomen and the skin is cut in the midline on the back of the head from the level of the eyes to the back of the neck. The skin is retracted and on one side the bone is cleaned by removing the muscle and connective tissue. A trephine hole is made about 1·5 cm. in front of the occipital crest and 1·0 cm from the midline. The hole is enlarged forwards and downwards with bone nibblers without damaging the venous sinuses which run into the dura mater below the occipital crest and in the midline. The hole should measure about 1·5 × 1·5 cm. and this should be large enough to allow the insertion of the decerebrating probe. Any bleeding which may occur from the bone is stopped with Plasticine or bone-wax. The dura mater is cut with fine sharp scissors and folded back over the edges of the hole in the skull. The flat probe is inserted and used to push the hemispheres forward so as to expose the midbrain. The midbrain is cut by pushing the blunt end of the probe downwards and forwards. The cerebral hemispheres are scooped out and the front of the cranium loosely filled with cotton wool. The skin on the scalp is now sewn or clipped together. The preparation should be left for half an hour for the anaesthetic to be blown off and for the blood clots to become firm. As with the spinal cat, the whole animal should not be given heparin for there is the risk of massive haemorrhage from the damaged vessels. To prevent clots forming in the arterial cannula, if the blood pressure is being recorded, twice the usual concentration of heparin should be present in the saline (p. 15).

The pithed animal. In a pithed animal the spinal cord has been destroyed and it is very suitable for testing pressor substances because it has an extremely low blood pressure[1]. It has also been used as a means of measuring the effects on blood vessels of stimulating the complete sympathetic outflow[2]. The animal which is usually employed is the rat and the preparation requires considerable skill and practice. Details are given on page 64.

[1] Shipley, R. E., Helmer, O. M. & Kohlstaedt, K. G. (1947). *Am. J. Physiol.*, **149**, 708.
[2] Gillespie, J. S. & Muir, T. C. (1967). *Br. J. Pharmac.*, **20**, 78–87.

Sterilization

In most of the experiments described in this book solutions and instruments do not need to be sterile because the animal is killed within a few hours at the most. This does not apply, however, to the experiments involving human subjects (pp. 60 and 76), to the guinea-pig wheal test (p. 34) and in the tests on behaviour in mice. In all these experiments it is necessary to use sterile syringes, needles and drug solutions.

Sterile disposable needles and syringes are convenient and cheap. If these are not available, needles and glass syringes may be sterilized by autoclaving them at 115° C. An ordinary household pressure-cooker is quite suitable, but the plunger of the syringe should be separated before sterilisation and re-assembled afterwards.

Sterile eye-drops and lamellae can be purchased but for methods of sterilizing other drug solutions a textbook of pharmaceutics[1, 2] should be consulted, because some drugs are unstable to heat and special methods must be used for sterilizing them.

[1] Gunn, C. & Carter, S. J. (1965). *Cooper and Gunn's Dispensing for Pharmaceutical Students*, 11th ed., pp. 400–535. London: Pitman Medical.

[2] Davis, H. (1961). *Bentley's Text-book of Pharmaceutics*, 7th ed., pp. 639–667. London: Baillière, Tindall & Cox.

Recording Devices—Mechano-electric Transducers[1]

For recording changes in length or tension, and changes in blood pressure, mechano-electric transducers of the 'resistance' strain-gauge type are frequently used. These gauges are wire strips or coils whose electrical resistance alters when they are stretched. The gauge is incorporated into one of the four arms of a Wheatstone bridge, across which a voltage must be applied (Fig. 18). At the start, the bridge is balanced by adjusting the resistance of one of the arms. When a force is applied to the strain gauge it will produce a change in resistance and a potential difference across the bridge. This is magnified by a DC amplifier and used to drive a recording potentiometer or galvanometer. Differential transformers are sometimes used instead. These are energized by AC voltages, and the output is measured with an AC amplifier. Both types of recording device are used and calibrated in similar ways.

Mercury manometers. For large animals, such as cats or rabbits, changes in blood pressure can be recorded with a simple U-tube, usually of 5 mm. bore, but for small animals the Condon-type manometer[2] (Fig. 19) is much more suitable. In this, the tubing is of narrow bore (2·5 mm.) and so the volume of fluid displaced into or out of the animal is small. In addition, the closed limb has a relatively wide bulb so the mercury level is altered very little even by quite large changes in pressure in the narrower open limb. The pressure can therefore be read directly because the zero is virtually constant.

Mercury manometers have the advantage that they are cheap, simple to use and give a direct reading with a wide excursion. Their disadvantages are their high inertia and the large volume of blood which may pass into or out of the animal with the possibility of clots forming in the cannula. With the Condon-type manometer the volume displaced is much smaller but there is still the problem of the high inertia of the system. With transducers, the volume changes are negligible and the system has low inertia, but they are expensive, more complicated to use, and do not give a direct reading. In addition the total width of the record is often only 5 cm.

[1] Lim, K. S. (1964). Transducers. In *Physical Techniques in Biological Research,* Vol. V, part A, chap. 6. Ed. Nastuk, W. L. New York: Academic Press.

[2] Condon, N. E. (1953) S.T.A. Bull., **3**, 9.

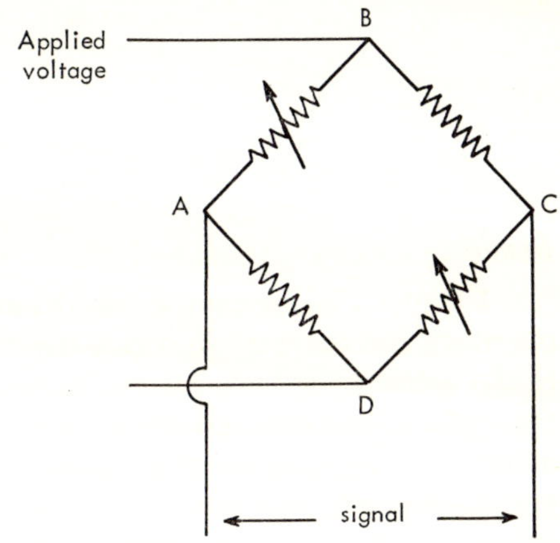

FIG. 18. Bridge circuit in a transducer. Four wire, or silicon semiconductor, units are arranged to form a Wheatstone bridge. The resistance of two of these, AB and DC, is altered by changes in tension, thus altering the potential across AC when a constant voltage is applied across BD. The use of matched units in all four arms of the bridge should prevent the balance being altered significantly by changes in temperature.

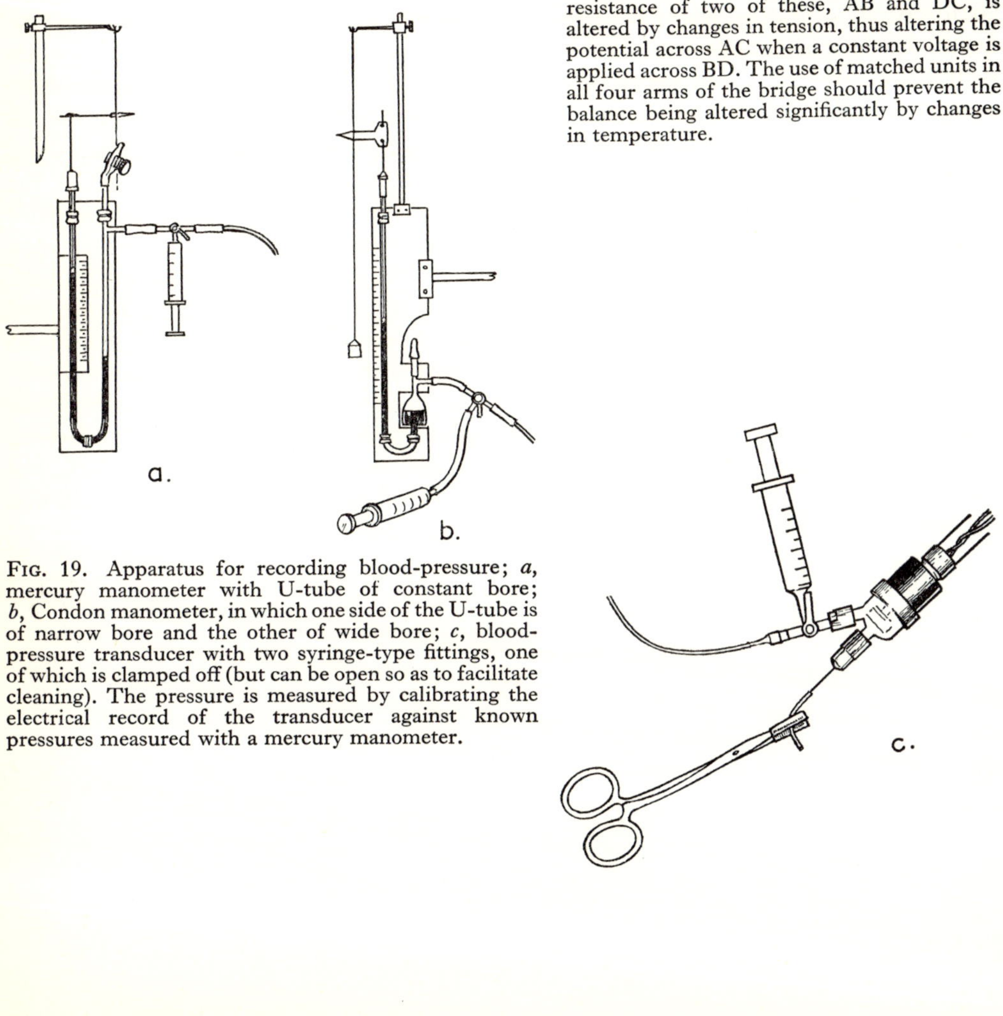

FIG. 19. Apparatus for recording blood-pressure; *a*, mercury manometer with U-tube of constant bore; *b*, Condon manometer, in which one side of the U-tube is of narrow bore and the other of wide bore; *c*, blood-pressure transducer with two syringe-type fittings, one of which is clamped off (but can be open so as to facilitate cleaning). The pressure is measured by calibrating the electrical record of the transducer against known pressures measured with a mercury manometer.

Results

Chapter 2 of the companion volume discusses the purpose of experiments in pharmacology and the ways in which the results can be compared qualitatively or quantitatively. In most experiments in this book graded responses are obtained, i.e. the size of the effect is variable and depends on the dose of the drug, so no new principles are involved in working out the results. In the experiment describing the testing of analgesics, however, the response is regarded as all-or-none. It is necessary to use groups of animals and to observe the proportion in which analgesia is detected, in order to calculate the dose of analgesic likely to produce analgesia in 50 per cent (ED_{50}). The principles involved are exactly the same as in assessing the results of an experiment to test the acute toxicity of a drug, in which the equivalent of ED_{50} is the LD_{50}, the dose which would kill 50 per cent of a group of animals. Although toxicity experiments are not included in this book, they are a very important part of pharmacology and have been described fully[1,2]. An outline of the theory is given in Appendix I.

[1] Finney, D. J., Goodwin, L. G. & Burn, J. H. (1952). *Biological Standardization.* London: Oxford University Press.

[2] Litchfield, J. T. & Wilcoxon, F. (1949). *J. Pharmac.* **96**, 99.

PREPARATIONS AND EXPERIMENTS

NOTE

Experiments and the Law in the United Kingdom

The Cruelty to Animals Act 1876 lays down that no experiment calculated to cause pain will be carried out on a living vertebrate animal unless subject to certain conditions. The most important of these are (i) that only experiments whose aim is the extension by new discovery of biological knowledge or knowledge useful for saving or prolonging life or alleviating suffering will be considered; (ii) that experimenters will be licensed; and (iii) the experiment will be carried out in a registered place.

If experiments are to be performed in illustration of lectures in medical schools, hospitals, colleges or elsewhere the demonstrator must hold, in addition to a licence, a Certificate C signed both by a Professor and a President of one of the Royal Societies named in the Act who certify that such experiments are absolutely necessary for the due instruction of the persons to whom such lectures are to be given with a view to their acquiring biological knowledge or knowledge useful to them in saving or prolonging life or alleviating suffering. Invariably attached to such a Certificate C are the conditions (i) that the animal will be anaesthetised throughout and (ii) that it will be killed before recovery from the anaesthetic.

Genuine experimental procedures, however, may be carried out either without an anaesthetic (Certificate A) or with an anaesthetic (Certificate B).

(i) *Without anaesthesia.* In this case a Certificate A signed by a Professor and President of one of the Royal Societies named in the Act, who certify that in their opinion insensibility in the animal in question cannot be produced by anaesthetics without necessarily frustrating an object of the experiment, is only allowed subject to the condition of limitation which requires that no operative procedure more severe than simple inoculation or superficial venesection may be adopted in any experiments under the Certificate A.

(ii) *With anaesthesia.* In any experimental procedure which exceeds the condition of limitation in severity the animal must always be anaesthetised, and for this the Certificate B is required to be signed by the statutory signatories who certify that the killing of the animal, on which the experimental procedure is performed, before recovery from the anaesthetic administered to it, would necessarily frustrate the object of the experiment. Recovery from the anaesthetic, i.e. survival of the animal, is thus permitted under Certificate B.

In all cases where the animal survives (i.e. under Certificate A or B) the whole procedures are strictly governed by the pain condition which at most does not permit severe pain which is likely to endure.

Survival procedures proposed on cats and dogs must be supported by an appropriate Certificate E (to support a Certificate A) and/or Certificate EE (to support Certificate B) in which the statutory signatories certify that the object of such an experiment will necessarily be frustrated unless permitted on an animal similar in constitution and habits to the cat or dog and that no other animal will avail. Such supporting Certificates E or EE are not required (for cats and dogs) in terminal or non-survival procedures (i.e. those covered by Licence Alone or by Certificate C); but in all cases, whether under Licence Alone or Certificates A, B or C, in which the horse, ass or mule is involved, a supporting Certificate F is required to be signed by the statutory signatories who certify that the object of such experiments will necessarily be frustrated unless it is performed on a horse, ass or mule and that no other animal will avail.

Any reference in this book to experiments, other than those carried out in illustration of lectures under Certificate C, applies to procedures which are exclusively experimental in the sense that their sole aim is to advance by new discovery biological knowledge or knowledge useful for saving or prolonging life or alleviating suffering. These procedures are mentioned in order to indicate how such genuine research projects can be carried out. Genuine research projects cover a very wide field including tests with new drugs.

DOSES

Although the doses quoted in this book are those usually found to produce an effect they do not always do so and may need to be increased or decreased by a factor of two or even more.

CHAPTER II

ACTIONS ON THE PERIPHERAL NERVOUS SYSTEM

1. NERVES

The most obvious effect which a drug can have on a nerve is to block the conduction of impulses along it. Usually sensory nerves are blocked more easily than motor nerves, and because drugs block sensation they are called local anaesthetics. Any substance which blocks sensory nerves, however, is likely also to block motor nerves if given in a high enough concentration.

The effects of drugs can be detected by showing the blockage in conduction (1) electrically, (2) by observing the disappearance of a reflex, or (3) in man, by observing the disappearance of sensation. Experiments with the first two types of method, using isolated preparations, have been described in Chapter 7 of the companion volume. To study effects in intact preparations the corneal reflex in rabbits[1] and the twitch-response of guinea-pig's skin[2] have been widely used. These tests can also be performed in man, though the corneal reflex test in man is normally only used qualitatively for demonstrating the effects of drugs, as in the experiment with drugs on the eye described on page 60. For the wheal test to be performed in man it is necessary to use the subject's sensation of pain, instead of the twitch-response of the animal. This method has been used to obtain accurate quantitative comparisons of local anaesthetics[3].

In the test using the corneal reflex, a solution of the drug is applied directly to the cornea and the time after this at which the corneal reflex disappears is noted. This time is inversely proportional to the rate of onset of anaesthesia. The relative activity of local anaesthetics can be estimated by comparing the concentrations which cause the blink reflex to disappear in about the same length of time. The result, however, is only a comparison of the rates of onset anaesthesia. Like the results obtained with the frog's sciatic plexus (described in the companion volume) these do not indicate differences in the duration or intensity of the effect. With the corneal reflex they are moreover complicated by the failure of certain drugs to cross mucous membranes.

With the twitch-response test in a guinea-pig's skin, an attempt is made to assess the duration and intensity of the effects, though it ignores differences in the rate of onset and in ability to cross mucous surfaces.

[1] Sollmann, T. (1918), *J. Pharmac.* **11**, 17.
[2] Chance, M. R. A. & Lobstein, H. (1944), *J. Pharmac.* **82**, 203; Bülbring, E. & Wajda, I. (1945), *J. Pharmac.* **85**, 78.
[3] Mongar, J. L. (1955), *Br. J. Pharmac.* **10**, 240.

The Guinea-pig Wheal Preparation

Guinea-pigs are prepared at least 24 hours before the experiment by first clipping and then shaving the hair on the lower back. A depilatory cream such as Veet can be used instead of shaving. Either method produces some irritation, but this generally disappears overnight. The sensitivity of the skin is greatest in the midline and slightly more in the upper part than in the lower part, consequently each concentration of drug must be tested in both areas. Two guinea-pigs each receive one dose in the front area and another in the back area (Fig. 20). Two other guinea-pigs receive the same two doses, but the solution which was used for the front is now used for the back; eight animals are therefore required to test two doses of two compounds (a, A and b, B). If the animals are large, however, it may be possible to make four injections in each.

To allow for variation in the sensitivity of the different parts of the skin and of different animals, the doses are given in all possible combinations:

	Front wheal	Back wheal
Guinea-pig 1	a	B
2	a	b
3	A	B
4	A	b
5	b	A
6	b	a
7	B	A
8	B	a

If four injections can be made in each guinea-pig, only four animals will be needed.

Intradermal Injection

A sterile sharp 26 G $\times \frac{3}{8}$ inch needle is used for each injection. The skin on the lower back of the guinea-pig is stretched taut by holding the animal with the hand placed around the abdomen and by pulling the skin taut with the thumb and forefinger (Fig. 21). The drug is injected in the same direction as that in which the skin is being held and the needle is inserted into the dermis or epidermis; considerable pressure is needed. If the plunger of the syringe is withdrawn slightly any appearance of blood indicates that the injection is subcutaneous, not intradermal, and it must be tried again. The volume injected (0·25 ml.) is enough to raise a wheal, which is outlined with a ball-point or felt-tipped pen. Five minutes after the injection the sensitivity of the area is tested by pricking with a needle, six times lightly, the skin at the site of injection and, as a control, the skin as far away from it as possible. Six twitches should be recorded for this control test, but the responses at the site of the injection will indicate the degree of anaesthesia, which is expressed as the number of negative responses, i.e. of failure to twitch; 6/6 indicates maximum anaesthesia and 0/6 indicates no anaesthesia. The test is repeated at five-minute intervals for a period of 30 minutes after the injection. The total score for

each wheal is added up and expressed as the total number of negative responses out of the 36 possible. The graph of log dose against effect is roughly linear in the middle part of the range, i.e. provided the doses are not so low as to be virtually ineffective or so high as to produce anaesthesia for the whole period of 30 minutes. The slopes of the lines for the two compounds can be compared and, if these are parallel, an equipotent molar ratio (or activity ratio) can be calculated by standard assay methods. If the pigs are big enough it may be possible to use four wheals with each, usually arranged left and right as well as front and back. The differences in sensitivity between left and right sides are smaller than between front and back, but the assay should be designed so that the doses are given equally to both sides as well as equally to front and back areas.

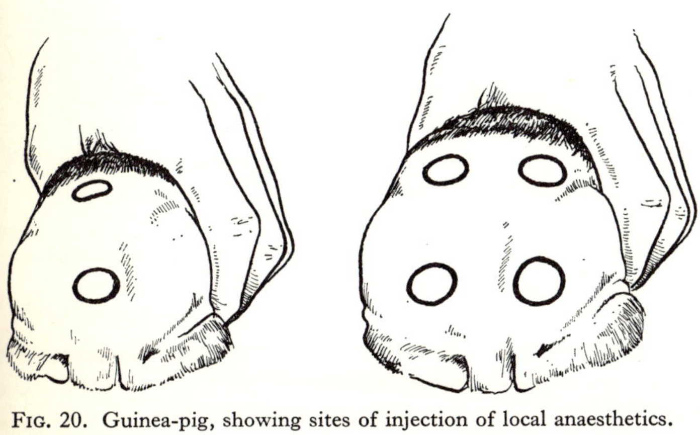

FIG. 20. Guinea-pig, showing sites of injection of local anaesthetics.

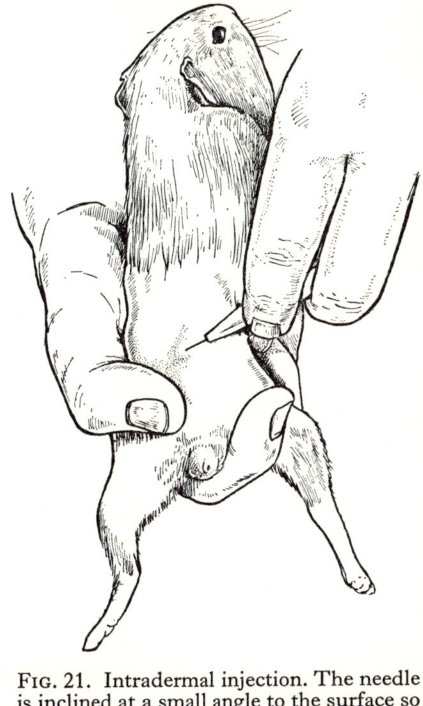

FIG. 21. Intradermal injection. The needle is inclined at a small angle to the surface so that it penetrates into the skin almost parallel to the surface and the injection can be made between the dermis and the epidermis.

Experiment 1 : A comparison of the local anaesthetic activity of procaine and lignocaine. Doses of 0·25 ml. procaine ($3{\cdot}33 \times 10^{-3}$ and 10^{-2} M) and of lignocaine (1·67 and 5×10^{-3} M), arranged as described above, are injected into at least two groups of eight animals, or one group if the animals are large and four injections can be made in each. It is wise to check that these concentrations are effective by testing two or three animals before starting. There is often a considerable variation in the sensitivity of different batches of guinea-pigs and the concentrations often require alteration by a factor of 2 either way.

Equipment required:

1. Electric clippers
2. Safety razor or depilatory cream (e.g. Veet or Immac)
3. Sixteen 26 G × 3/8 inch sharp hypodermic needles
4. Several 1 ml. tuberculin syringes
5. A fine felt-tipped pen
6. A stop watch or time clock
7. Several darning needles.

Solutions required:

1. Procaine hydrochloride, $3{\cdot}33 \times 10^{-3}$ M (or 1 mg. procaine hydrochloride/ml.).
2. Procaine hydrocholride, 10^{-2} M (or 3 mg. procaine hydrochloride/ml.).
3. Lignocaine hydrochloride, $1{\cdot}67 \times 10^{-3}$ M (or 500 μg. lignocaine hydrochloride/ml.).
4. Lignocaine hydrochloride, $5{\cdot}0 \times 10^{-3}$ M (or 1·5 mg. lignocaine hydrochloride/ml.).

N.B.—The solutions should be made up in 0·9 per cent saline and be sterile.

The pH of the solution will affect the result and should be measured carefully and adjusted to 7·4 if necessary.

Time required: The experiment takes about 2 to 2½ hours to perform by a group of four people; about this amount of time is also required on the previous day for two people to prepare the guinea-pigs.

Notes. In addition to the big differences in the sensitivity of guinea-pig skin, the results of this experiment are often markedly affected by differences in the skill with which the intradermal injection is made and, to a lesser extent, by differences in the method for testing the reflex. Although the time taken to perform the experiment is reduced by increasing the number of people involved, the accuracy of the result may be considerably reduced too.

It will be found that the graphs of log dose against degree of anaesthesia for the two drugs are not parallel and their relative activity can only be expressed as a range. Students should study the variance of their estimates of the mean score for the various doses and see which of them, if any, are significantly different. Compare the results with those on isolated preparations (Experiment 30 in the companion volume). Other drugs which may be used are: cocaine (try $6{\cdot}0 \times 10^{-4}$ and $1{\cdot}8 \times 10^{-3}$ M), amethocaine (try $3{\cdot}33 \times 10^{-4}$ and $1{\cdot}0 \times 10^{-3}$ M) and cinchocaine (try $2{\cdot}0 \times 10^{-4}$ and $6{\cdot}0 \times 10^{-4}$ M).

2. THE NEUROMUSCULAR JUNCTION

Note. Special permission is required from the Home Office for testing neuromuscular blocking agents in animals, even when they are anaesthetized, and 48 hours' notice of an experiment must be given to the local inspector. These regulations do not apply, however, to spinal or decerebrate animals, kept under artificial respiration; legally speaking these animals are dead.

In the companion volume several isolated preparations are described for testing the effects of drugs which interfere with transmission at the neuromuscular junction. Unless the muscles are very thin, however, they cannot be kept *in vitro* for any length of time. In addition, the results may be complicated by the need for drugs to diffuse into their site of action so that substances of high molecular weight may appear to be very slow-acting. To study the effects of drugs on preparations of any size it is necessary to retain the blood supply, i.e. to use an intact preparation, and to inject the drug intra-arterially, as close to the muscle as possible.

The Cat Tibialis Preparation[1]

Induction

A cat is anaesthetized with nitrous oxide 4 parts, oxygen 1 part, and halothane 3 to 4 per cent (p. 19). Other methods of induction can be used, but this one causes least distress. When the animal is unconscious and flaccid, the front of the neck is shaved with electric clippers or the fur cut off with scissors. The trachea is exposed and cut and a glass cannula is inserted and firmly tied in place (p. 16). If an anaesthetic machine with a 'Cyclator' is available the anaesthetic gases can be administered through this direct to the trachea. If this machine is not available the trachea is connected to a Woulfe's bottle containing ether (p. 20). The animal may now be spinalized or decerebrated (p. 24), or deep prolonged anaesthesia can be produced by a slow intravenous injection of chloralose 40 to 80 mg./kg.

Anaesthesia with chloralose. Chloralose is not particularly soluble in saline and to obtain a 1 per cent solution it must be heated to about 80°C. before it will dissolve, and allowed to cool to 40°C. before injection into the animal. The temperature is fairly critical because, if the solution is too cold, chloralose will crystallize out in the syringe or venous cannula. It is advisable to start preparing the solution before anaesthetizing the animal and to allow it to cool during the dissection. Alternatively, the chloralose may be dissolved in a mixture of polyethyleneglycol and water, 50 per cent v/v. At room temperature it is soluble in concentrations up to $2\frac{1}{2}$ per cent so that between 1·6 and 3·2 ml. of solution are injected per kg. This is a smaller volume than that needed if the warm solution in saline is used.

[1] Brown, G. L. (1938), *J. Physiol.* **92**, 22P.

Either of the femoral veins or of the cephalic veins is suitable for the intravenous injection of the chloralose. The femoral vein is located by feeling the pulse from the femoral artery on the inside of the groin. The skin is shaved and lifted and an oval piece about $1\frac{1}{2} \times 2\frac{1}{2}$ cm. is cut out with scissors. The femoral vein is seen, together with the artery and nerve, below a thin layer of connective tissue (Fig. 22). The cephalic vein can be seen when the skin on the inside of the lower forelimb is removed (Fig. 23) and great care is needed when exposing it because the vein is very near the surface. Either of these veins is cannulated with a plastic cannula made from tubing about 1·5 mm. in diameter with the tip drawn out to about 1 mm. (p. 14). The other end of the cannula is connected to a three-way tap and the whole unit is filled with saline. To stop any clot forming in the tip of the cannula a small amount of heparinized saline (p. 15) is injected, so as to fill the cannula up to the tip, but not enough to enter the animal in any quantity and cause bleeding during the rest of the dissection.

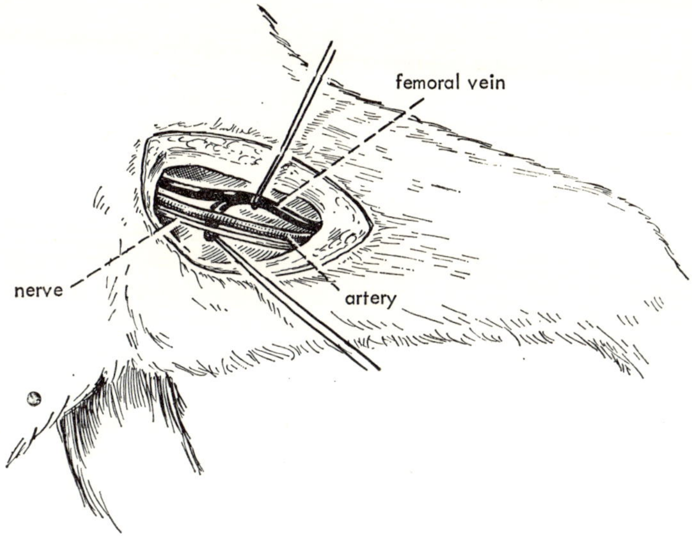

FIG. 22. Location of the femoral vein.

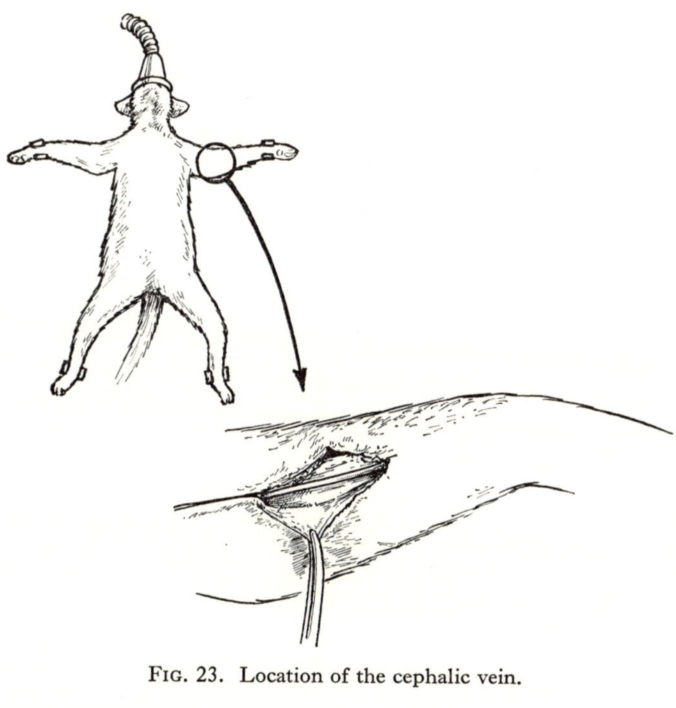

FIG. 23. Location of the cephalic vein.

Preparation of the Carotid Artery (Fig. 24)

The carotid artery is located together with the vagus nerve and superior cervical ganglion immediately under a longitudinal bundle of muscle which runs parallel to, and just beside, the trachea. The artery is separated from the nerve trunk and freed from connective tissue, so that a length of about 2 to 3 cm. is obtained. A loop of thread is placed around it, but it is better to cannulate at a later stage so that injection of the heparin can be delayed until after the dissection.

Preparation of the Nerve (Fig. 25)

The right leg is more convenient to use. The rump and the whole of the leg are shaved. The skin from the protuberance of the ischial tuberosity on the buttock is cut with sharp scissors almost to the back of the ankle, so as to obtain access to the popliteal space. This is opened with the fingers to expose the sciatic nerve, which is seen as a large trunk dividing into the medial and lateral popliteal nerves. A strong thread is passed around the main sciatic nerve high in the popliteal space, and tied tightly to sever any central connections. The lateral popliteal nerve, complete with the sheath containing the blood supply, is dissected free from the surrounding connective tissue and a pair of platinum electrodes is applied and protected with cotton wool, liquid paraffin and Parafilm (Fig. 26). The medial popliteal nerve is cut or tied, and the popliteal space closed by sutures or clips in such a way that the electrode is held firmly in place between the sutured edges.

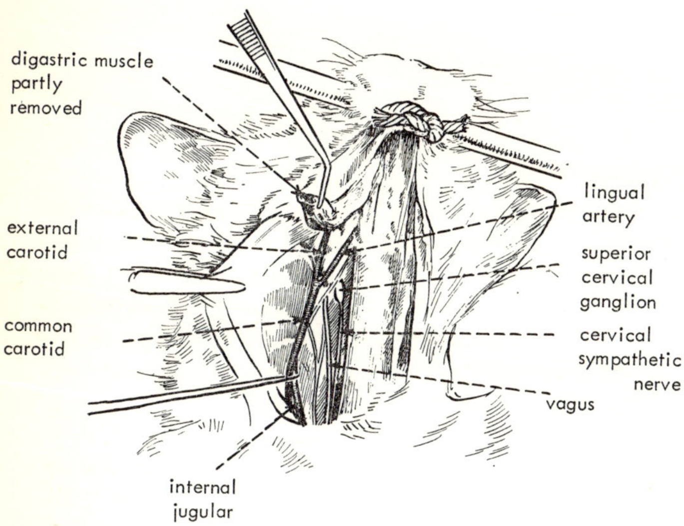

FIG. 24. Location of the carotid artery and vagus and cervical sympathetic nerves.

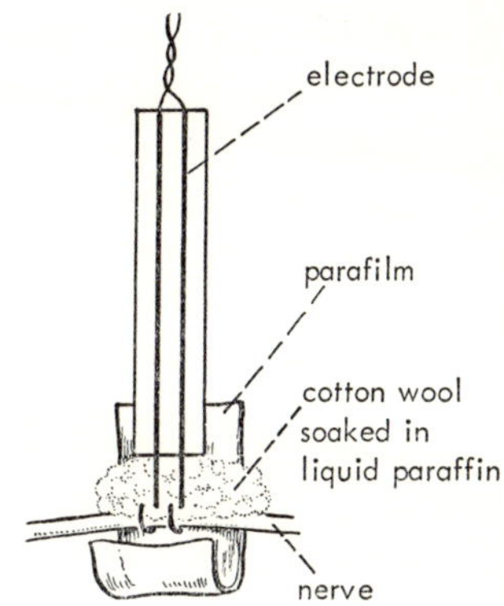

FIG. 26. Attachment of lateral popliteal nerve to electrodes.

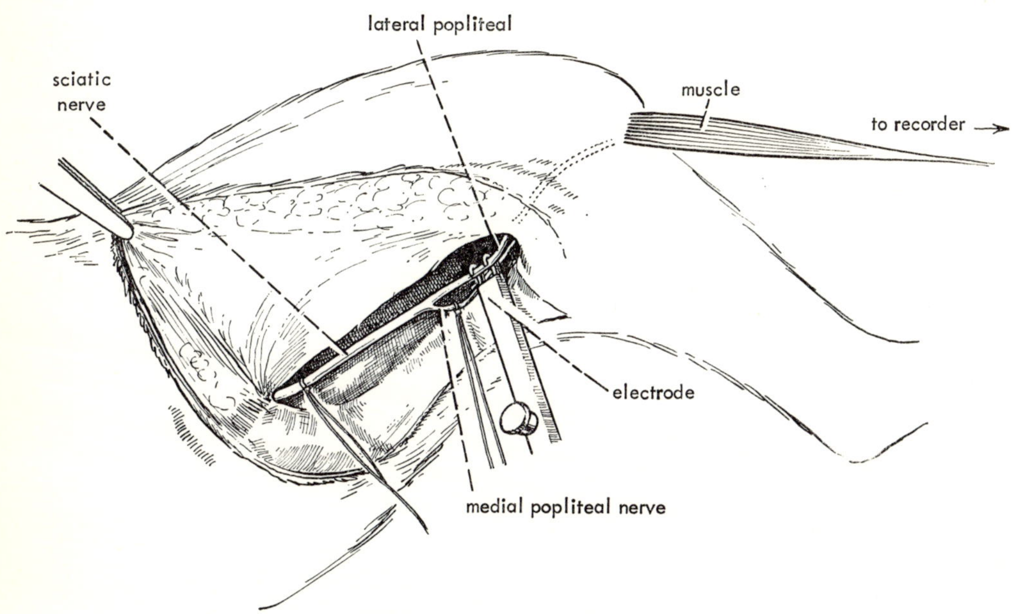

FIG. 25. Location of the lateral popliteal nerve (which leads to the anterior tibial nerve). *Note.* The lateral popliteal nerve has also been called the peroneal nerve.

Preparation of the Muscle (Fig. 27)

The tibialis muscle runs beside the tibia, and its tendon passes through a band of ligaments to cross over the front of the ankle and become inserted on a knob of bone on the inside of the foot. An incision is made from this knob along the front of the leg nearly to the knee. Care is needed because there are several large vessels just under the skin, some of which must be tied off. The transverse ligament, located just above the ankle joint, is cut and the insertion of the tendon together with the bony knob attached to it is cut off. Bone clippers or ordinary finger-nail clippers are suitable for cutting the bone. The hole is dried and sealed with Plasticine or fibrin dust. The tendon is then dissected free up to the belly of the tibialis anterior muscle. The belly of the muscle is freed from its envelope of connective tissue and all exposed tissue is moistened with liquid paraffin to minimize dehydration. The anterior tibial artery should now be visible, lying posterior to the belly of the muscle. It is generally quite small, being about 1 mm. in diameter, but occasionally it can be larger. The artery is freed for a distance of about 2 cm. just proximal to the ankle joint and a thread is placed around it. If desired, the fine branches to the extensor longus digitorium can be tied and this muscle removed, and then the branches leading to the peroneal group of muscles can be tied. This step takes time however, and can well be omitted.

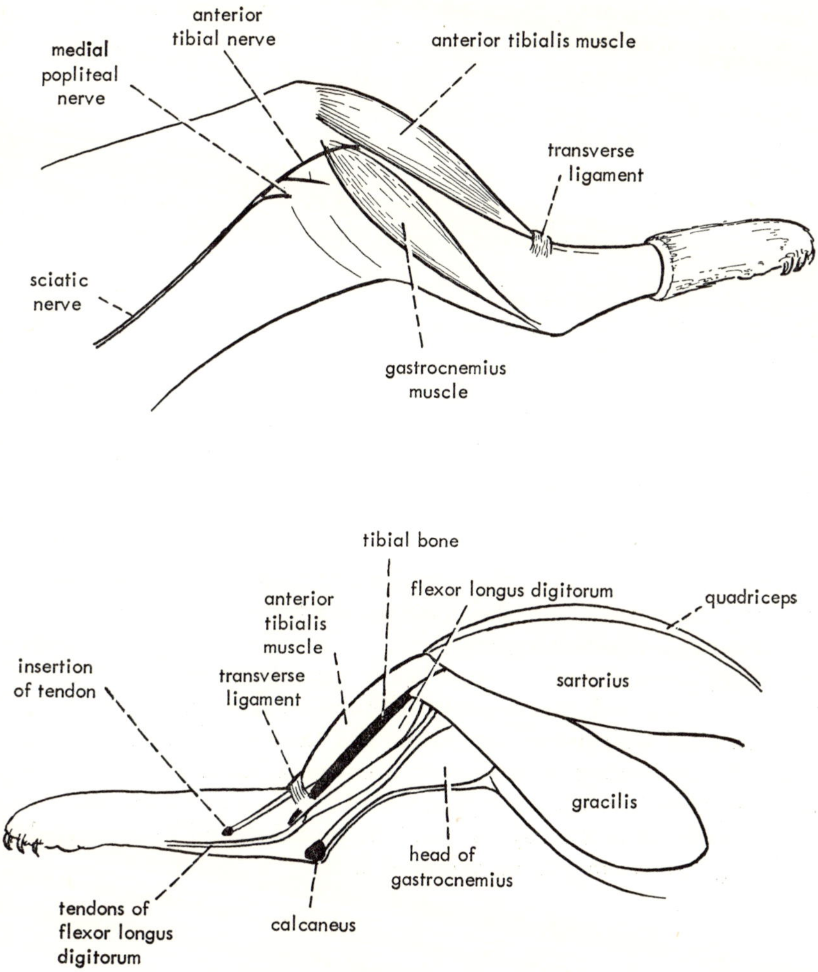

FIG. 27. Anatomy of the cat's leg.

A length of strong linen or silk thread (gauge 1) is tied around the end of the tendon; the bony knob is used to prevent the tie slipping off. The extensor tendons to the foot are cut and the limb fixed to a Brown-Schuster myographic stand (C. F. Palmer, London) by drill bars (Fig. 28). The smaller drill goes from the inside of the leg at right angles into the lower end of the tibia. The larger drill goes into the condyles of the femur. These operations can be performed easily by using a bradawl to make guide holes and pushing the drills by hand in with a minimum of turning, to ensure a firm grip. It is important to make sure the drills are approximately at right angles to the leg and parallel to each other.

With the animal on its back and the limb flexed, the drills are fitted into the myographic stand. The tibia is fixed in a horizontal position for use with a strain gauge, or in the vertical position if the flat spring on the myograph is to be used. The foot is tied out of the way and the skin sutured above the muscle. A layer of gauze soaked in liquid paraffin is applied to the exposed area. The thread tied to the tendon is attached to a strain gauge (max. working range ca. 1 to 2 kg./mm.) or to the myograph spring holding a lever writing on a smoked drum.

Cannulation of the Anterior Tibial Artery

A small bulldog clip or a remote control clamp (Fig. 29) is applied to the anterior tibial artery and a fine plastic cannula is inserted and firmly tied in place. The cannula is attached to a suitable injection apparatus (e.g. Fig. 12) which allows injection of the drug followed by a saline wash-in. Just before cannulation 0·3 to 0·6 ml. of heparin (5,000 units/ml.) is injected intravenously. The carotid artery is now cannulated with a plastic cannula filled with heparinized saline and the blood pressure recorded with a mercury manometer writing on a smoked drum or a blood-pressure transducer and electrical amplifier and recorder; a typical record is shown in Figure 30.

The preparation is now ready for use. The animal should be supported with sand bags and the leg kept warm with an overhead lamp.

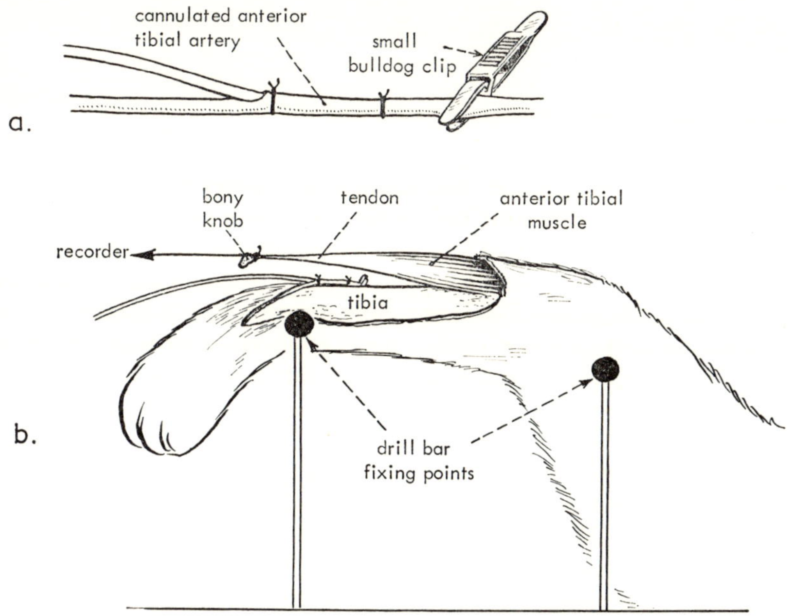

FIG. 28. Cat tibialis preparation, showing *a*, cannulation of the anterior tibial artery and *b*, the points of inserting the drill bars to fix the hind limb.

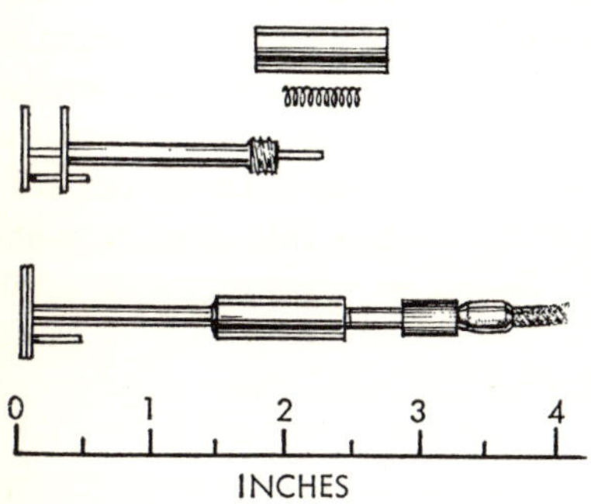

FIG. 29. Remote-control clamp.

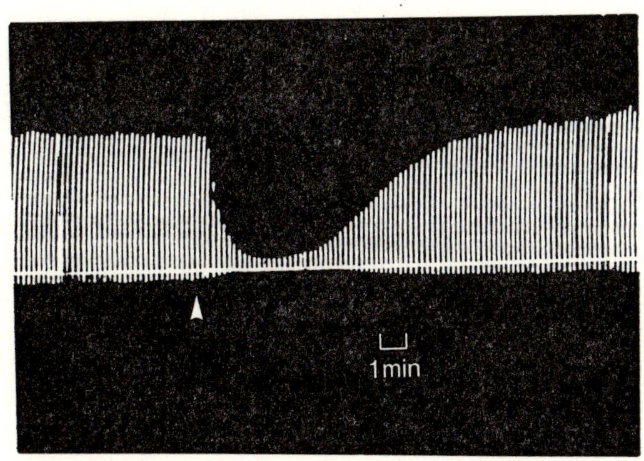

FIG. 30. Contractions of the tibialis muscle of the cat in response to electrical stimulation of the peroneal nerve once every 10 seconds. A neuromuscular blocking agent was injected at the arrow.

Experiment 2: Drugs and the neuromuscular junction. Test the response of the tibialis muscle to stimulation of the sciatic nerve with 0·5 m-sec. pulses, at a frequency of 1 every 10 sec. The initial intensity of stimulation should be less than 3 volts and the voltage should then be gradually increased until a maximal twitch response is obtained. The voltage is then increased by about a further 50 per cent to ensure that the stimulus is supramaximal. When drugs are being given close arterially the nerve stimulation is stopped and resumed a minute later.

1. Observe the effect of a close arterial injection of 0·3 ml. saline. If no response is obtained, make a rapid injection of acetylcholine 40 to 80 nanomoles (10 to 20 μg. acetylcholine bromide) and wash it in with 0·2 ml. saline. Compare the 'twitch' obtained with that produced by the close arterial injection of similar amounts of carbachol and of 100 micromoles of potassium chloride (7·45 mg.) washed with 0·2 ml. saline. Observe the effects of a tetanus by stimulating the nerve for 6 sec. at a rate of 50 pulses/second.

2. Inject suxamethonium, 40 nanomoles (15 μg. of suxamethonium chloride, $2H_2O$, 20 μg. suxamethonium bromide, $2H_2O$) intra-arterially and observe both its immediate effects and its subsequent effects on the responses to nerve stimulation.

3. When the preparation has fully recovered, observe the effects of the intravenous injection of (+)-tubocurarine chloride in doses of from 20 to 200 nanomoles (15 to 150 μg. (+)-tubocurarine chloride). When a fairly steady block of neuromuscular conduction is achieved, test the response of the muscle to a tetanus and to the close arterial injection of acetylcholine and/or potassium chloride as in (1) above. Observe the effects on the block produced by (+)-tubocurarine chloride of the intravenous injection of neostigmine, 30 to 60 nanomoles (10 to 20 μg. neostigmine bromide), or physostigmine, 100 nanomoles (30 μg. physostigmine sulphate). Gallamine triethiodide, 20 to 200 nanomoles (18 to 180 μg.), maybe used instead of, or as well as, (+)-tubocurarine chloride.

4. When the preparation has fully recovered and the control responses to nerve stimulation and to the intra-arterial injection of acetylcholine are normal, observe the effects of the intravenous injection of decamethonium, 100 nanomoles (50 μg. decamethonium iodide). When a fairly steady block of neuromuscular conduction is achieved, test the response of the muscle to a tetanus and to the close arterial injection of acetylcholine and potassium chloride as in (1) above. Also observe the effects of the intravenous injection of the same dose of neostigmine or physostigmine as was used in (3).

5. When the preparation has fully recovered and the control responses to nerve stimulation and to the intra-arterial injection of acetylcholine are normal, observe the effects of (–)-nicotine, 200 to 400 nanomoles (100 to 200 μg. nicotine di(hydrogen-tartrate), $2H_2O$).

6. If the preparation still continues to give satisfactory responses, observe the effects of the intravenous injection of triethylcholine iodide, 40 nanomoles (12·5 μg. triethylcholine iodide). At a low rate of stimulation, some degree of block usually occurs in about 10 min. and is maximal after 20 min. Test the effects on this block of a tetanus and the close arterial injection of acetycholine and potassium chloride as in (1) above. Also observe the effects of a dose of (+)-tubocurarine chloride as in (3). The block may eventually be reversed by the slow intravenous injection of choline chloride, 100 μmoles (15 mg. anhydrous choline chloride).

Solutions required: The doses to be used in this experiment are suitable for a medium sized animal (1 to 2 kg.). They must be injected in a small volume of saline (0·1 ml.) and this volume should be the same for all injections. It is therefore convenient to have relatively strong stock solutions of drugs which can be diluted as required; e.g. if a solution of (+)-tubocurarine 10^{-3} M is diluted 2 ml. to 10 ml. with saline, 0·1 ml. of the diluted solution (2×10^{-4} M) will contain 20 nanomoles (15 μg. of (+)-tubocurarine chloride B.P.) The following strengths of stock solutions (in 0·9 per cent saline) are suggested with this idea in mind:

1. Suxamethonium, 3×10^{-3} M (or 1·5 mg. suxamethonium bromide, $2H_2O$/ml.).
2. Decamethonium, 10^{-2} M (or 5 mg. decamethonium iodide/ml.).
3. (+) – Tubocurarine, 10^{-3} M (or 1 mg. (+) – tubocurarine chloride, $5H_2O$/ml.).
4. Gallamine triethiodide, 10^{-3} M (or 1 mg. gallamine triethiodide/ml.).
5. Acetylcholine, 10^{-3} M (or 200 μg. acetylcholine chloride/ml.).
6. Carbachol, 10^{-3} M (or 200 μg. carbachol chloride/ml.).
7. Physostigmine, 10^{-2} M (or 3 mg. physostigmine sulphate/ml.).
8. Neostigmine, 3×10^{-3} M (or 1 mg. neostigmine bromide/ml.).
9. Potassium chloride, 10^{-1} M (or 7·5 mg. potassium chloride/ml.).
10. (–) – Nicotine, 10^{-2} M (or 5 mg. (–) – nicotine di (hydrogen tartrate)/ml.).
11. Triethylcholine, 3×10^{-3} M (or 500 μg. triethylcholine iodide/ml.).

Time required: The preparation takes at least two hours to set up and the testing of drugs may last all day.

It is unwise to attempt both (5) and (6), as the effects of (–)-nicotine last for a very long time.

Equipment required:

1. A Brown-Schuster myograph apparatus with fixation drills (C. F. Palmer, London).
2. A kymograph and smoked drum or a force-displacement transducer with amplifier and electrical recorder.
3. A mercury manometer or a blood-pressure transducer with amplifier and electrical recorder.
4. An anaesthetic mask or an anaesthetic machine.
5. A respiration unit or a 'Cyclator', for ventilation of the animal.
6. A heated operating table and overhead operating lamp.
7. Tracheal, venous and arterial cannulae.
8. An injection block or some similar method for injecting drugs and for allowing a saline wash-in.
9. A small flat stimulating electrode.
10. A stimulator.
11. Electric clippers.
12. Bone cutters or large nail clippers.
13. Sutures and a curved suture needle.
14. Retractor hooks and clips.
15. Skin clips (not essential).
16. A bradawl.
17. Gauze and cotton wool.
18. Liquid paraffin.
19. Parafilm.

Notes. Note the differences in the time courses of suxamethonium, (+)-tubocurarine and nicotine.

The block produced by (+)-tubocurarine is antagonized by cholinesterase inhibitors, but the block produced by depolarizing agents is deepened by the addition of cholinesterase inhibitors. Sometimes an initial supramaximal contraction is seen with drugs which produce a block by first causing a depolarization.

Other nerves and muscles have been used, e.g. the sciatic nerve and the gastrocnemius or quadriceps muscles and the femoral nerve and the sartorius or gracilis muscles (Fig. 27). These differ considerably in their sensitivity to drugs like decamethonium but the tibialis nerve-muscle preparation has been the most widely used.

3. AUTONOMIC GANGLIA

In the companion volume there are descriptions of a number of isolated preparations of smooth and cardiac muscle, which can be used to study the effects of drugs on certain parts of the autonomic nervous system. They do not include, however, preparations involving sympathetic ganglia. Although isolated preparations containing these structures have been described[1], it is usually more convenient to work with a preparation which has its normal blood supply intact. The superior cervical ganglion preparation of the cat, described below, also has the advantage that the response to preganglionic stimulation is a contracture of the nictitating membrane, which can be recorded mechanically; there is no need to dissect out the post-ganglionic nerve so as to record the response electrically though this can be done if desired.

The Cat Superior Cervical Ganglion Preparation[2, 3]

A cat is anaesthetized and tracheal and femoral cannulae are inserted exactly as in the cat tibialis preparation (p. 37).

Preparation of the Femoral Artery (Fig. 31)

Because the superior cervical ganglion is situated in the neck, it is not convenient to use the carotid artery to record the blood pressure and the femoral artery is used instead. The femoral artery of the leg not used for the intravenous injections is exposed and cleared of connective tissue for a distance of about 2 cm. A loop of 1/0 thread is placed around it in preparation for cannulation after the ganglion has been prepared.

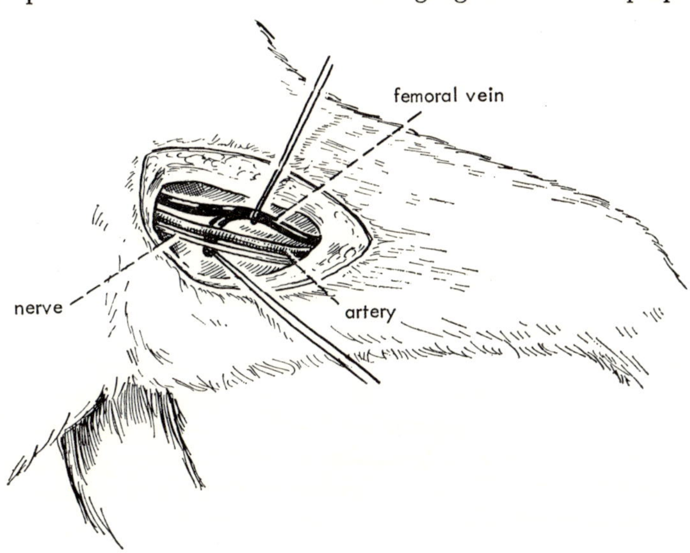

FIG. 31. Location of the femoral artery.

[1] Quilliam, J. P. (1959). *Br. J. Pharmac.*, **14**, 277–283.
[2] Paton, W. D. M. & Perry, W. L. M. (1953). *J. Physiol.*, **119**, 43–57.
[3] Trendelenberg, U. (1954). *Br. J. Pharmac.*, **9**, 481–487.

Preparation of the Nictitating Membrane (Fig. 32)

A strong fine thread (preferably of silk or nylon which does not stretch) is sewn through the nictitating membrane. Take care to see that it does not occlude the vein running round the edge! Usually the right membrane is chosen but either may be used, whichever is the more convenient for exposing the preganglionic nerve and arterial blood supply to the ganglion.

Dissection of the Nerve and Blood Supply (Fig. 33)

The head is immobilized by securing the jaws to a transverse rod. The front of the neck is presented for dissection by tying the arms tightly to the sides of the animal and placing a 'pillow' under the nape of the neck. The common carotid artery is found under two muscle bundles (the sternohyoid and the sternomastoid) running parallel to the trachea. Alongside the common carotid is the small internal jugular vein and a large nerve trunk which consists of the vagus nerve and the cervical sympathetic nerve. The latter is the preganglionic nerve supplying the superior cervical ganglion and during the rest of the dissection this nerve, which is dissected out later, should not be pulled or allowed to dry out.

The skin on the front of the neck is cut with scissors in the midline from the tracheal cannula towards the muzzle, until a transverse vein is seen lying under a thin layer of connective tissue. This vein is ligated and cut. The common carotid artery is followed from where it is exposed near the tracheal cannula up to where the lingual artery branches from the external carotid. Blunt dissection must be used for this because the area is very vascular. A large nerve (the hypoglossal) passes over the area where the carotid artery divides and must be separated from the arteries. The lingual artery is much smaller than the carotid and curves inwards towards the trachea. The external

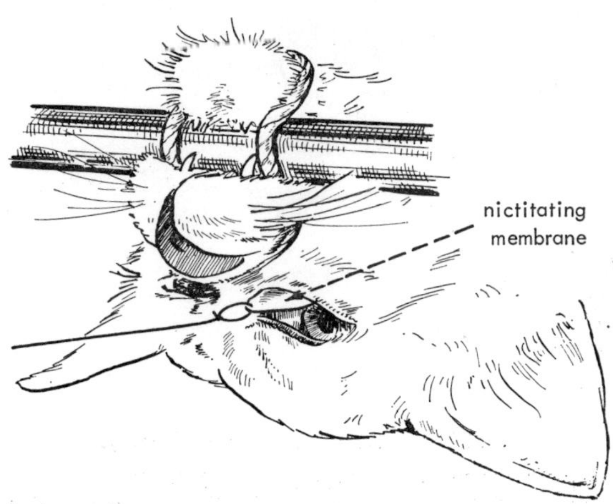

FIG. 32. The cat's nictitating membrane.

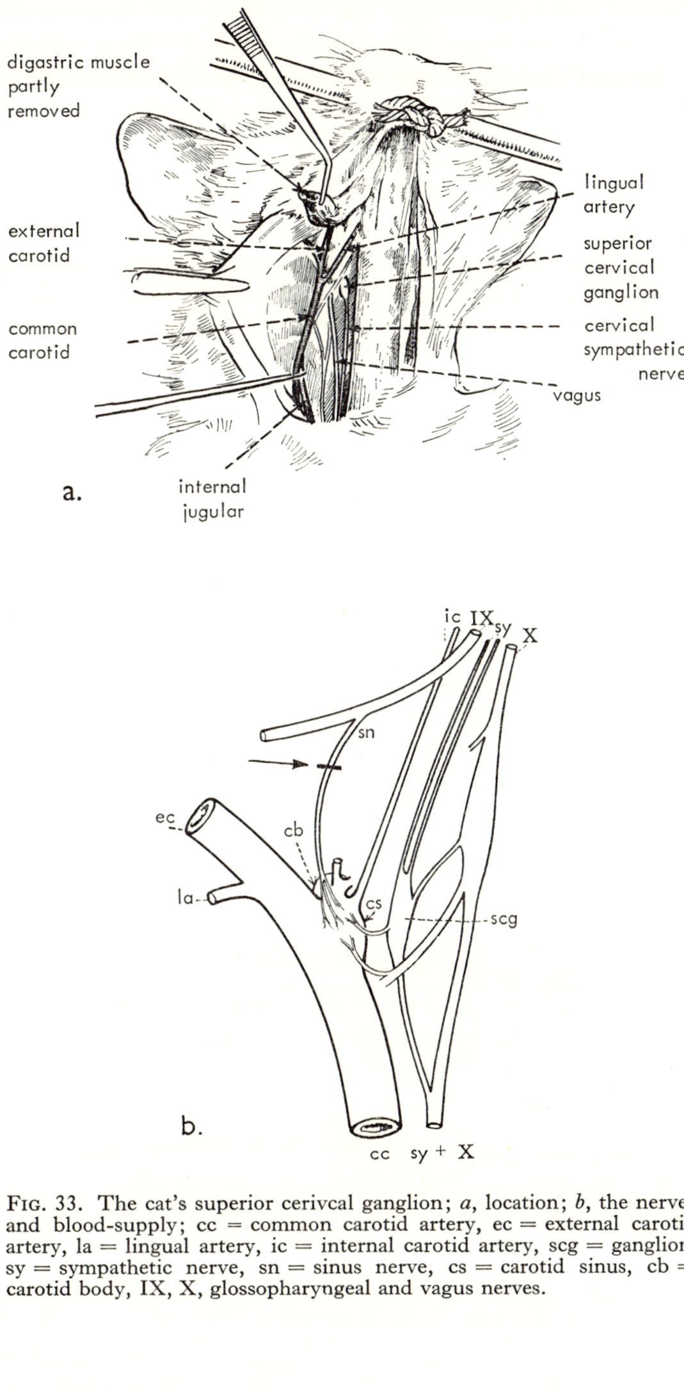

FIG. 33. The cat's superior cerivcal ganglion; *a*, location; *b*, the nerves and blood-supply; cc = common carotid artery, ec = external carotid artery, la = lingual artery, ic = internal carotid artery, scg = ganglion, sy = sympathetic nerve, sn = sinus nerve, cs = carotid sinus, cb = carotid body, IX, X, glossopharyngeal and vagus nerves.

carotid curves downwards and outwards, towards the animal's face. The lingual artery is more accessible, but it is smaller and more difficult to cannulate than the external carotid. The latter artery can be exposed by removing a bundle of muscle (the digastric) lying over the top of it and it is sometimes also necessary to remove a large lymph gland. The large blood vessels of these two pieces of tissue should be tied before their removal.

Different methods can be used for arranging the preparation for the injection of drugs. In one (A) the drug is injected retrogradely into the ganglion; in another (B) the drug can be injected either retrogradely into the ganglion or into the blood supply to the nictitating membrane. The methods differ in that in A the external carotid is tied, whereas in B it is only clamped and if the injection (into the lingual artery) is made slowly with the clamp off, the effects of the drug on the postganglionic receptors in the nictitating membrane should be seen.

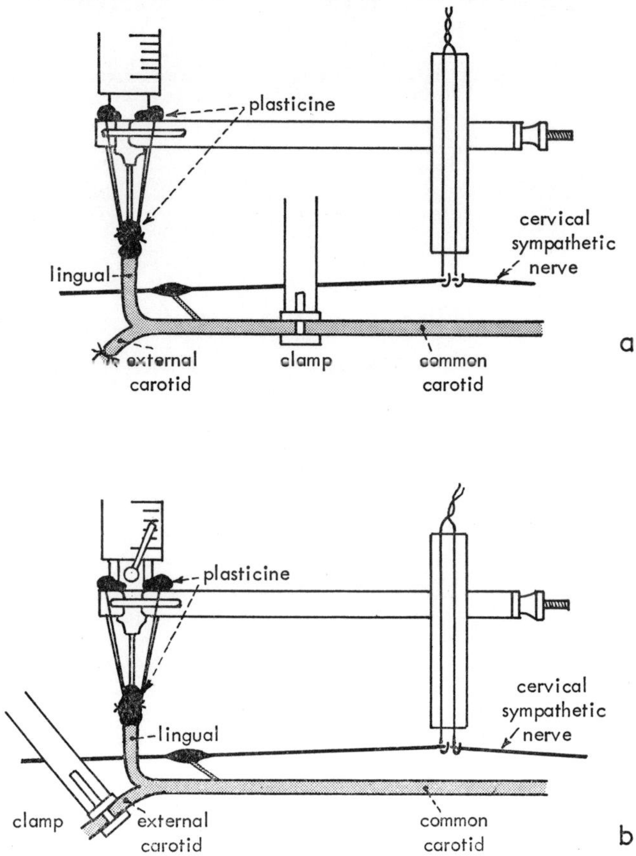

FIG. 34. Cannulation of the lingual artery; *a*, with external carotid tied off; *b*, alternative arrangement with clamp on external carotid which is applied when injections are made.

Cannulation of the artery

A. The artery (lingual or external carotid) is dissected free from connective tissue for a distance of at least 1 cm. from the common carotid. Two fine ligatures are firmly tied close together around the distal portion of the artery, but the threads are not cut off. Another ligature is tied 2 to 3 mm. more distal still and the artery is completely severed between the first two and the third tie. The threads of the third tie are cut off. A stump of artery, about 1 cm. in length, with four threads attached to it is thus obtained. An adapted Luer-lock hypodermic needle is held in a thermometer clamp and this is positioned with an X-block immediately over the arterial stump. The X-block is tightened enough to make the thermometer clamp firm, but still loose enough for it to be swung up or down a few centimetres. A 1 ml. tuberculin syringe filled with saline is attached to the needle which is then also filled with saline. To prevent clotting 0·3 to 0·6 ml. of heparin, 5,000 units/ml., is injected intravenously. A remote controlled bulldog clamp (p. 45) is placed on the extreme end of the common carotid just before it divides into the external carotid and the lingual arteries. The end of the arterial stump is cut as for cannulation, and the end of the adapted hypodermic needle is inserted. The four threads are attached to the end of the thermometer clamp with Plasticine and the artery is tied firmly to the needle. The X-block holding the thermometer clamp is then firmly tightened. It is probably advisable to try to cannulate the lingual artery and if this is not successful the external carotid is used instead. When one has been successfully cannulated the other is tied off (Fig. 34*a*).

B. If the lingual artery has been cannulated and the external carotid artery has not been tied off, it is possible to arrange to make injections either to the blood supply to the ganglion or to the blood supply to the nictitating membrane itself by placing the remote controlled bulldog clamp on the carotid artery just beyond the junction with the lingual artery (Fig. 34*b*). If the clamp is applied and the injection made rapidly into the lingual artery, most of the drug passes retrogradely into the circulation to the ganglia. If the clamp is not applied and the injection made slowly (over a period of 6 to 8 sec.) the drug will pass into the circulation to the nictitating membrane and none should pass into the circulation to the ganglion. A tap must be inserted between the syringe and the needle cannula, however, to prevent the arterial blood pressure forcing the plunger out of the syringe and to allow it to be filled.

Recording

The thread which has been attached to the nictitating membrane can now be passed over a pulley and attached to a lightly sprung lever which has a magnification of 10 and a load of 5 g. writing on a smoked drum. Alternatively it is attached to an amplifier and electrical recorder and to a force-displacement transducer (max. working range of 0·2 kg./mm.) mounted upon a horizontal adjustment screw. The tension on the thread is adjusted until the pen deflection reads 5 g. on a previously calibrated scale on the paper.

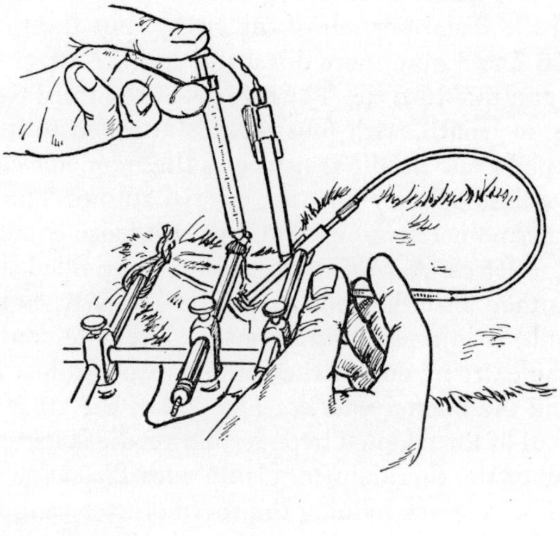

C.

FIG. 34*c*. General view of arrangement for holding syringe, remote-controlled bulldog and electrodes.

Stimulating the Preganglionic Nerve

The vago-sympathetic trunk, which has previously been exposed, is carefully dissected out and the preganglionic sympathetic nerve (the smaller of the two) is separated with great care and placed over a pair of platinum electrodes which are held in position by a clamp. The nerve is protected with liquid paraffin, cotton wool and 'Parafilm' (Fig. 26). It is stimulated with rectangular wave pulses of 0·7 m.-sec. duration at a rate of 10 shocks per second. Usually a stimulus of 3 to 5 volts will produce a maximal contracture of the membrane. When stimulant drugs are being tested, electrical stimulation is used to test if the ganglion is still transmitting, or whether it has been fully or partly blocked by the frequent application of stimulant drugs. When blocking agents are being tested the preganglionic nerve is stimulated maximally and continuously and the degree of relaxation of the membrane is used as a measure of the blocking activity of the drug.

Cannulation of the Femoral Artery

The femoral artery, which has been exposed previously, is cannulated and the blood pressure recorded by any of the methods described on p. 18. Although the animal has already received heparin when the lingual or external carotid artery was cannulated, it is still advisable to have heparinized saline in the cannula in the femoral artery.

Close Arterial Injection

A. The saline in the needle head is sucked out with a syringe and the space filled with drug solution and a syringe containing the drug dissolved in 0·1 ml. of saline is fitted. If the lingual (or external carotid) artery has been cannulated and the external carotid (or lingual) artery has been tied off, the remote controlled clamp on the common carotid artery is momentarily released and the drug rapidly injected. An injection of 0·2 ml. saline is given in between doses of drugs and repeated if there is any response from drug solution left in the cannula.

B. If the cannula is placed in the lingual artery and the external carotid artery has not been tied off, it is necessary to apply the clamp during the injection (instead of releasing it) to ensure that the drug reaches the ganglion, first opening the tap between the syringe and the needle cannula (and shutting it after the injection!). If the clamp is not applied and the injection is made slowly, over a period of 6 to 8 sec., the drug will reach the nictitating membrane but not the ganglion. Stimulant drugs can be injected every 5 to 10 min. but sometimes the effects of blocking drugs last for a long time. A typical record is shown in Figure 35.

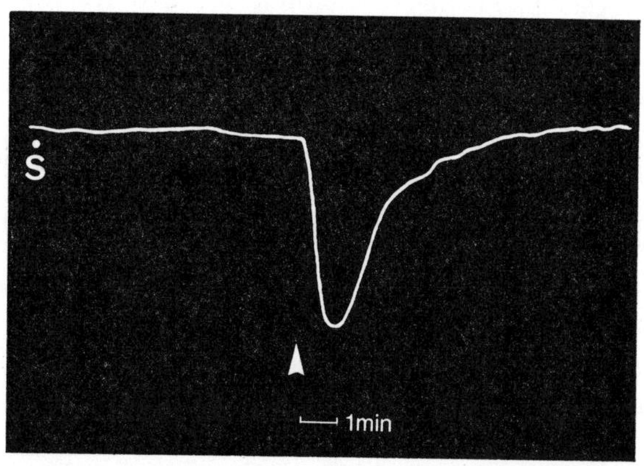

FIG. 35. Contracture of the nictitating membrane of the cat caused by continuous stimulation of the sympathetic nerve. A ganglion-blocking agent was injected at the arrow.

Experiment 3 : Drugs and the superior cervical ganglion and nictitating membrane. Stimulate the preganglionic nerve with supramaximal pulses (see Experiment 2) at a rate of 10/sec. for 10 sec. Observe the effects of the injection of 0·2 ml. saline with and without stimulation of the preganglionic nerve.

Without stimulating the nerve, investigate the effects of doses of:

1. Acetylcholine, 40 to 200 nanomoles (10 to 50 μg. acetylcholine iodide).
2. Dimethylphenylpiperazinium (DMPP), 10 to 20 nanomoles (3 to 6 μg. DMPP iodide).
3. Pilocarpine, 100 to 200 nanomoles (25 to 50 μg. pilocarpine nitrate).
4. (−)-Nicotine, 10 to 40 nanomoles (5 to 20 μg. nicotine di(hydrogen tartrate), $2H_2O$).
5. Histamine, 10 to 30 nanomoles (3 to 9 μg. histamine di(hydrogenphosphate)).

Stimulate the preganglionic nerve continuously and test the ganglion blocking effects of doses of:

6. Hexamethonium, 500 nanomoles to 2·5 μmoles (150 to 750 μg. Hexamethonium bromide).
7. (−)-Nicotine, 75 to 100 nanomoles (40 to 50 μg. nicotine di(hydrogentartrate), $2H_2O$).
8. (+)-Tubocurarine chloride, 5 to 10 nanomoles (4 to 8 μg. (+)-tubocurarine chloride B.P.).
9. Atropine, 30 nanomoles (10 μg. atropine sulphate).

If the preparation has been cannulated so that drugs may be injected either into the circulation to the nictitating membrane or to the ganglion, it is also possible to investigate the effects, without stimulating the preganglionic nerve, of doses of:

10. Noradrenaline, 5 to 50 nanomoles (1·5 to 15 μg. noradrenaline hydrogentartrate, H_2O) (a) on the nictitating membrane and (b) on the ganglion.
11. Acetylcholine as in 1 above on the nictitating membrane.
12. Noradrenaline as in 10 after the intravenous injection of guanethidine, 20 μmoles (5 mg. guanethidine sulphate).

Solutions required: As in Experiment 2, the doses indicated are for a medium sized cat (about 2 kg.). It is necessary to prepare stock solutions of drugs which can be diluted so that the effective dose is present in 0·1 ml.

1. Acetylcholine, 5×10^{-3} M (or 1 mg. acetylcholine iodide/ml.).
2. Dimethylphenylpiperazinium, 5×10^{-4} M (or 200 μg. DMPP iodide/ml.).
3. Pilocarpine, 5×10^{-3} M (or 1·5 mg. pilocarpine nitrate/ml.).
4. (−)-Nicotine, 5×10^{-3} M (or 2·5 mg.(−)-nicotine di(hydrogen) tartrate)/ml.).
5. Histamine, 5×10^{-4} M (or 1·5 mg. histamine di(hydrogen phosphate)/ml.).
6. Hexamethonium, 5×10^{-2} M (or 20 mg. hexamethonium bromide/ml.).
7. (+)-Tubocurarine, $2{\cdot}5 \times 10^{-4}$ M (or 200 μg. (+)-tubocurarine chloride/ml.).
8. Atropine, 10^{-3} M (or 400 μg. atropine sulphate/ml.).
9. Noradrenaline, 5×10^{-4} M (or 100 μg. noradrenaline hydrogen tartrate/ml.).
10. Guanethidine, 2×10^{-1} M (or 100 mg. guanethidine sulphate/ml.), which does not require further dilution.

Equipment required:

2 to 11, 13 to 15, 17 to 19 as for Experiment 2.
plus

20. Bench clamps, rods, X-blocks for assembly to hold animal's head and the other accessories (see Fig. 34).
21. Arterial cannula made from a 18 to 20 gauge Luer-lock hypodermic needle.
22. Thermometer clamp to hold 21.

Time required: The preparation takes 2 hours to set up and will then last for several hours though it does not last as long if the external carotid is tied off as it does if it is only clamped off when injections are made into circulation to the ganglia.

Notes. This experiment should show clearly the effects of ganglion-stimulants and of ganglion-blocking drugs. It should also show that it is possible to stimulate the ganglion with some drugs, such as histamine and pilocarpine (also with 5-hydroxytryptamine) which are not blocked by hexamethonium. If the cannulation has been arranged so that drugs can be injected either to the ganglion or to the nictitating membrane, it should be possible to show that noradrenaline does not affect the ganglion and that acetylcholine does not act directly on the nictitating membrane. The preparation can be used to study adrenergic blocking agents and drugs such as guanethidine which interfere with the release of noradrenaline.

The Chronically Denervated Nictitating Membrane

For this preparation the superior cervical ganglion on one side of the cat has been excised under general anaesthesia and aseptic conditions two to three weeks before the experiment. This allows the eye on the side of the lesion to develop maximal supersensitivity to sympathomimetic drugs.

Under pentobarbitone anaesthesia, dissect the superior cervical ganglion on the intact side, and cut its post-ganglionic nerves. Prepare both nictitating membranes for the recording of tension, as in the previous experiment. It is advantageous to use a force transducer here rather than a lever because control over the amplification enables one to correct for the considerable differences between the tensions developed by the two nictitating membranes in response to a single dose of drug. Also prepare a vein for the injection of drugs and a femoral artery for recording arterial pressure.

Determine the threshold doses of adrenaline and noradrenaline for both nictitating membranes. Then construct dose/response curves for both drugs on both membranes. Using the acutely denervated membrane as control, compare the supersensitivity developed by the chronically denervated membrane for adrenaline with that developed for noradrenaline.

The preparation can be used for the differential assay of mixtures of adrenaline and noradrenaline.

If facilities for aseptic surgery with recovery are not available, partial supersensitivity can be induced by 'pharmacological denervation' of one nictitating membrane. This can be done by instilling guanethidine eye drops daily into one eye for three weeks. Both nictitating membranes can then be acutely denervated in the course of the experiment.

4. THE HUMAN EYE

The human eye is far too valuable to be a suitable object for testing new drugs, unless these have been very thoroughly studied in animals first. Moreover, it is not really suitable for quantitative comparisons. It can, however, be conveniently and safely used for showing, qualitatively, the effects of many drugs which act at sites on the autonomic nervous system. The changes which can be observed are:

1. in the size of the pupil,
2. in the ability to focus the eye,
3. in reflex responses,
4. in the conjunctival vessels.

1. The size of the pupil can be measured by a pupilometer (Fig. 36). This consists of a card with pairs of pin holes punched in it. At one end the holes are 8 mm. apart; at the other they are 2 mm. apart. Between these extremes, the adjacent pairs of holes differ in spacing by 0·5 mm. The subject closes one eye and, holding the card close to the other eye, looks through the holes at a distant object, which should be well illuminated. The object is to find a pair of holes through which the images appear just to be touching each other. The distance between these holes is taken as a measure of the pupil diameter. If the holes are further apart than the pupil diameter, a space will appear between two images, if they are closer together than the pupil diameter, the two images will appear to merge.

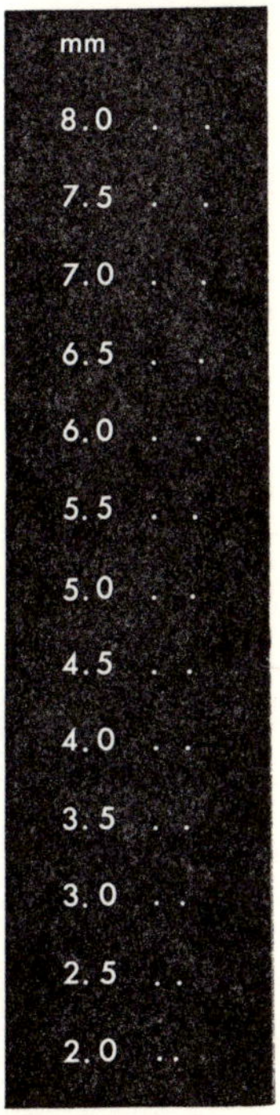

FIG. 36 The pupilometer.

2. The ability to focus the eye can be measured with Snellen's printed charts. To assess distant vision the subject is placed 6 metres from a standard type chart and a note is made of the smallest type which can be read without error. Each size of type is numbered, with a large number indicating large type which should be legible at a large distance. The row of type marked D6 should be legible at 6 metres. If only type of size D15 can be read at 6 metres the visual acuity is 6/15. Drugs which impair distant vision will, therefore, be seen to decrease the visual acuity ratio.

To assess near vision 'small type' cards are used, held 30 cm. from the eye. Again a note is made of the smallest type which can be read without error but this is used directly as a measure of the acuity. The numbers on these cards increase in size with decreasing size of type, the opposite of the arrangement on the charts used for distant vision, but in both situations impairment of vision is indicated by a decrease in number.

The near point is also measured. The subject notes the smallest type he can read when a small type card is 30 cm. away. The card is then brought progressively closer and a note is made of the distance (in cm.) at which the type can still be read.

3. Effects on reflex responses can be studied by using a wisp of cottonwool to test the corneal reflex and by shining a bright light into the eye to test the light reflex. It is important that the person testing the corneal reflex should stand at the side of the subject and not in front of him. The wisp of cottonwool should be applied from the side so that the subject is as little aware as possible of its approach. It should lightly brush the cornea and not touch the eyelid or eyelashes. When testing the light reflex it is important to shade the eye for at least 30 sec. beforehand.

The effects of drugs on the reflex can only be described qualitatively. Usually they are almost all or none, i.e. the reflex is either blocked or unaffected.

4. The effects on the conjunctival vessels, likewise, can only be assessed qualitatively, but should indicate the vasoconstrictor or vasodilator properties of drugs to some extent.

Experiment 4: Drugs and the human eye. Investigate the effects on pupil size, distant vision, near vision, near point, corneal reflex, light reflex and conjunctival vessels, of the following:

Cocaine hydrochloride, 3·8 micromoles, 1·3 mg.
Ephedrine sulphate, approximately 10 micromoles, 2 mg.
Physostigmine salicylate, approximately 50 nanomoles, 0·02 mg.
Pilocarpine nitrate, approximately 2 micromoles, 0·5 mg.
Homatropine hydrobromide, approximately 500 nanomoles, 0·2 mg.

Only one drug should be tested in each subject and there should be at least one observer for every two subjects. Long-sighted people should not be given homatropine because they are likely to have a higher intraocular pressure than normal and homatropine may raise it further. After control readings have been made, the drug is applied to the eye and the readings repeated 10, 20 and 30 minutes later. Cocaine, physostigmine and homatropine can conveniently be administered as lamellae, i.e. gelatin discs containing the drug, if these are obtainable. Note that for physostigmine and homatropine only a quarter of the lamella is used. These are picked up with the slightly moistened end of a camel-hair brush. Ephedrine sulphate and pilocarpine nitrate are applied as drops of solution (about 0·1 ml.) from a dropper. The person administering the drug should stand at the side of the subject who should look straight ahead. The eyelids are held apart with the forefinger and thumb of one hand and the lamella or drop of drug solution is applied to the cornea with the other hand. If the subject is approached from the side there is much less likelihood that he will blink; he is sure to blink if approached from the front. The untreated eye may be used as an additional control for studying effects on reflexes and on the conjunctival vessels but may not be very satisfactory for the effects on accommodation, because there are usually considerable differences between the visual powers of the two eyes.

The effects of the drug may last for several hours but not as long as overnight. Subjects should be warned not to drive a car whilst their vision is affected. If the effects of homatropine are severe, physostigmine may be given as an antidote, but this is seldom necessary.

Apparatus required: Test type cards for distant and near vision, ruler, pupilometer, torch, cottonwool.

Drugs required: Lamellae containing cocaine hydrochloride (1·3 mg.), physostigmine salicylate (0·065 mg.) and homatropine hydrobromide (0·65 mg.). The lamellae of physostigmine and homatropine should be divided into quarters. If lamellae are not obtainable an equivalent amount of sterile solution of the drug must be used instead.

Solutions required: Solutions containing ephedrine sulphate (20 mg./ml., approx. 10^{-1} M), pilocarpine nitrate (5 mg./ml., approximately 2×10^{-2} M).

The drug solutions should be sterilized; standard ophthalmic preparations should be used if possible.

Time required: With five subjects and three observers the experiment can be completed in one hour, though the subjects' vision may not return to normal for up to 12 hours.

Notes. The local anaesthetic properties of cocaine should clearly be seen, also its ability to potentiate the effects of sympathetic stimulation. Note its effect on pupil size and on the conjunctival vessels. Compare its action with those of ephedrine.

With physostigmine, pilocarpine and homatropine, effects will be observed on accommodation as well as on pupil size. Compare the results obtained with ephedrine and with homatropine.

CHAPTER III

THE CARDIOVASCULAR SYSTEM

Drugs acting on the cardiovascular system are traditionally characterized by their effects on blood pressure—hence the classification into pressor and depressor actions. These actions can provide extremely sensitive means for the biological assay of drugs, and examples of preparations suitable for this purpose are given here.

Such preparations are of little or no value, however, in the elucidation of a drug's actions on the cardiovascular system. A drug can influence blood pressure by actions on the flow of blood through the systemic vascular bed or by actions on the resistance of that bed. The resistances of two parts of the vascular bed may be changed in opposite directions, with a consequent increase in flow through one region and a decrease through another. Since most organs require flow rather than pressure, a drug that raises blood pressure by vasoconstriction may be harmful where a drug giving rise to a similar pressure change by increasing flow would be beneficial. An increase in flow through the circulation can itself be due to a primary action on the heart, or to a primary action on the capacity vessels, raising the venous filling pressure of the heart.

If the blood pressure and cardiac output are measured simultaneously it is possible to apply the equation,

$$\text{Peripheral resistance} = \frac{\text{blood pressure}}{\text{cardiac output}}$$

and thus to characterize drugs as 'overall vasoconstrictors' or 'overall vasodilators'. This is rather a futile exercise, however, as it ignores the elasticity of blood vessels, and the possible effect of drugs on the capacity of the circulation. If a drug raises the cardiac output, the resulting pressure rise will passively distend the arterioles and thus reduce their resistance. The fallacy of this approach is illustrated by the experiment of injecting a constrictor drug into the splenic circulation, which has a high ratio of capacity to resistance. Contraction of the spleen raises the venous pressure and hence the cardiac output. The increased arterial pressure will cause a marked fall in the peripheral resistance and may even increase the blood flow through the constricted splenic arterioles.

In order to study the sites of action of a drug on the cardiovascular system it is thus necessary to design experiments so that either pressure or flow is under control.

Preparation of Animals for recording Blood Pressure

1. *Anaesthetized Rats*

Anaesthesia. A rat (200 to 300 g.) is anaesthetized with urethane 0·6 ml./100 g. (0·3 ml. intraperitoneally and 0·3 ml. subcutaneously) of a 25 per cent w/v solution in water, 1 hour before the experiment. Amylobarbitone sodium, 100 mg./kg. can be injected intraperitoneally instead of urethane, but it does not produce the same prolonged anaesthesia.

The animal is placed on its back on the operating table, the legs are fastened, and the head is pinned down (Fig. 37). The trachea is exposed and cut (p. 16) and a glass or plastic cannula is inserted and firmly tied in place. A retaining thread is attached to prevent the cannula from slipping out. There is sometimes an accumulation of mucus in the trachea and this can be removed either with a feather or with a twisted piece of cottonwool passed down the cannula into the trachea. It is important that the bronchioles and lungs are not damaged because this will cause oedema and can lead to respiratory problems. The common carotid artery is located in the neck. It lies together with the vagus and the cervical sympathetic nerves and the small internal jugular vein in the space between a lateral bundle of muscle, the longus capitis, and the trachea. It is easily exposed by separating the two muscle bundles, the sternomastoid and sternothyroid, which lie above it. The artery is separated from the nerves and vein and carefully freed of connective tissue. A thread is placed around it but it is not cannulated at this stage.

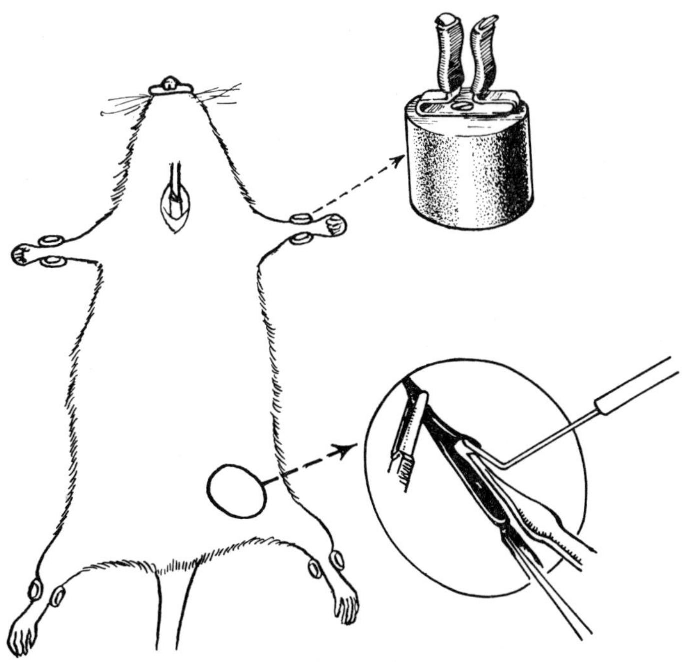

Fig. 37. The anaesthetized rat, showing clamps for paws and (inset) cannulation of the femoral vein.

Cannulation of the vein (Fig. 37). The venous cannula can be inserted into an external jugular vein (one on the opposite side to the carotid artery which has been chosen) or into either of the femoral veins. There are many branches of the jugular vein which need to be tied off and it is often more convenient to use a femoral vein, even though it is smaller. A piece of skin about 1 × 2 cm. is cut free from the inguinal region close up by the abdominal wall. The subcutaneous fat is carefully 'torn' away, with two forceps, exposing a vein leading to the skin. This is tied and cut. The femoral vein is then exposed and the portion between the junction with the saphenous vein and the inguinal ligament is very carefully cleared free of connective tissue. A small vein which enters dorsally from the thigh muscle must be located and tied off, with fine thread (No. 5/0) but not cut. If this is not done there will be 'bleeding back' during the cannulation. A fine plastic cannula (1·5 mm. external diameter drawn out to 0·25 to 0·5 mm.) is connected to an injection block (Fig. 12) which allows injection of the drug followed by saline to wash it all in. With this method there is a minimum dead space involved. The whole unit is filled with heparinized saline (p. 15) and all air bubbles are excluded. A fine bulldog clip is put on the vein close to the abdominal wall and the vein distended (p. 16). The vein is tied at its junction with the saphenous vein and this leaves about 1 to 1½ cm. of distended vein ready for cannulation. A slight tension is placed on the vein (p. 17). It is cannulated and the bulldog clip can be removed, and the cannula pushed in a further centimeter and firmly tied in place (do not crush it).

Cannulation of the artery. The carotid artery can now be cannulated. To prevent clots, 0·05 to 0·1 ml. of heparin (5,000 units/ml.) is injected intravenously through the cannula already inserted and washed in with 0·2 ml. of saline. A plastic cannula, slightly larger than the venous cannula (p. 14) is connected to a Condon mercury manometer or a blood-pressure transducer and the whole unit filled with heparinized saline, taking care to exclude all air bubbles. The cannula is inserted and the clamps are removed after the unit has been tested for leaks (p. 18). It is more convenient to use a blood-pressure transducer and here again the exclusion of all air bubbles is essential.

Note. It is sometimes necessary to put the animal on artificial respiration (p. 21) and it is important that the rate and volume of the ventilation is correct. Rats are particularly sensitive to over-inflation or ventilation at too fast a rate, which cause oedema of the lungs.

2. *Pithed Rats*[1,2]

A rat is anaesthetized with sodium pentobarbitone (p. 21) injected intraperitoneally and the trachea cannulated so that ventilation can be maintained artificially. The animal also receives heparin, but only a small dose, 0·05 ml. (5000 units/ml.) because there is more injury to tissues in the preparation of the pithed rat than in the anaesthetized rat and so greater risk of excessive bleeding with large doses of heparin. One carotid artery is prepared for cannulation, as described for the anaesthetized rat (p. 63) and the other carotid artery and the two jugular veins are tied off. The pithing rod should be about 2 mm. in diameter and 25 cm. long, with one end bluntly pointed;

[1] Shipley, R. E., Helmer, O. M. & Kohlstaedt, K. G. (1947). *Am. J. Physiol.*, **149**, 708; Shipley, R. E. & Tilden, J. H. (1947). *Proc. Soc. exp. Biol. Med.*, **64**, 453–455.

[2] Gillespie, J. S. & Muir, T. C. (1967). *Br. J. Pharmac.*, **30**, 78–87.

it can be made from stiff wire. The rat's head is held taut and in line with the vertebrae, with the thumb in the middle of the angle on the mandible, and the forefinger across the top of the skull. The point of the pithing rod is inserted obliquely into and through the eye socket at an angle of about 45° to the long axis of the rat. After the skull has been entered, the rod is aligned with the vertebral column and passed through the cranium and thence down the whole length of the spinal canal. It is advisable to leave the pithing rod in place because withdrawing it often causes bleeding. The carotid artery is now cannulated and connected to the blood-pressure recorder as in the anaesthetized rat preparation.

3. *Anaesthetized Cats*

Anaesthesia is induced in the cat by one of the methods described on page 18 and a decerebrate, spinalized or anaesthetized animal may be used. For testing depressor drugs it is advisable to use an anaesthetized preparation, which has a relatively high blood pressure. In the decerebrate and spinal preparations the blood pressure is much lower and they are more suitable for testing pressor drugs. The blood pressure can be recorded from the femoral artery (p. 54), but it is generally more convenient to use one of the carotid arteries, as described on page 64. For the injection of drugs the femoral vein is usually exposed and cannulated (p. 38) though the cephalic vein (p. 38) may be used instead. The animal is given heparin (0·3 to 0·6 ml. of 5,000 unit/ml.) as usual and left for about 10 minutes before any drugs are injected. Typical records of the blood pressure are shown in Figure 38.

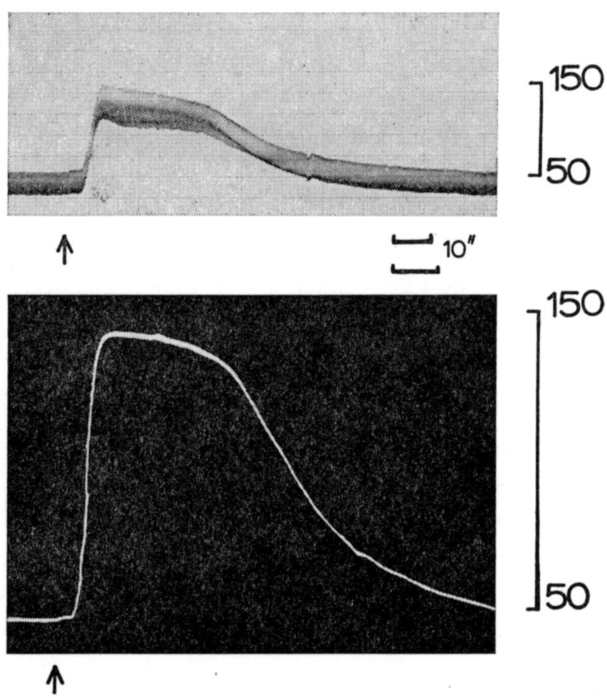

FIG. 38. The rise in blood-pressure in an anaesthetized rabbit produced by adrenaline, injected intravenously at the arrow. The upper trace was obtained with a transducer connected to one femoral artery and the lower trace with a mercury manometer connected to the other femoral artery. Note that the mercury damps the pulse-pressure. The lines on the right-hand side show the calibrations in mm. Hg; the kymograph was moving slightly faster than the pen-recorder.

Experiment 5 : Effects of drugs on the blood pressure of the anaesthetized rat. Observe the effects of the intravenous injection of the following, the doses being dissolved in 0·1 to 0·2 ml. saline and washed in with 0·2 ml. saline:

1. 0·2 ml. saline.
2. (–)-Adrenaline, 3 nanomoles (1 μg. adrenaline hydrogen tartrate BP).
3. (–)-Noradrenaline, 3 nanomoles (1μg. noradrenaline hydrogen tartrate).
4. (±)-Isoprenaline, 1 nanomole (0·3 μg. (±)-isoprenaline sulphate BP).
5. Acetylcholine, 2·5 nanomoles (0·5 μg. acetylcholine iodide).
6. (–)-Nicotine, 50 nanomoles (25 μg. nicotine dihydrogen tartrate, $2H_2O$).
7. Atropine, 500 nanomoles (200 μg. atropine sulphate BP) or oxyphenonium, 50 nanomoles (20 μg. oxyphenonium bromide).
8. Repeat 5, 2, and 6.
9. Acetylcholine, 25 to 250 nanomoles (5 to 50 μg. acetylcholine iodide).
10. Hexamethonium, 5 μmoles (2 mg. hexamethonium bromide).
11. Repeat the highest dose used in 9, repeat 6, 2 and 3.
12. Ergotoxine, 300 nanomoles (200 μg. ergotoxine ethane sulphonate).
13. Repeat 2, 3 and 4.
14. Propranolol, 350 nanomoles (100 μg. propranolol hydrochloride).
15. Repeat 2, 3 and 4.
16. Histamine, 2 nanomoles (0·6 μg. histamine dihydrogen phosphate BP).
17. Posterior pituitary extract (vasopressin), 0·05 units.

Time required: It takes about 1 hour to set up the preparation and about 2 hours to test the effects of the drugs.

Solutions required: The doses indicated are for a medium-sized rat (200 to 250 g.). The following stock solutions should be prepared and the dose required is present in 0·1 ml.

1. 0·9 per cent sodium chloride.
2. 3×10^{-5} M adrenaline (or 10 μg. adrenaline hydrogen tartrate/ml.).
3. $3{\cdot}0 \times 10^{-5}$ M noradrenaline (or 10 μg. noradrenaline hydrogen tartrate, H_2O/ml.).
4. 10^{-5} M isoprenaline (or 3 μg. isoprenaline sulphate, H_2O/ml.).
5. $2{\cdot}5 \times 10^{-5}$ M acetylcholine (or 5 μg. acetylcholine iodide/ml.).
6. $2{\cdot}5 \times 10^{-3}$ M acetylcholine (or 0·5 mg. acetylcholine iodide/ml.).
7. 5×10^{-4} M (–)-nicotine (or 250 μg. (–)-nicotine dihydrogen tartrate, $2H_2O$/ml.).
8. 5×10^{-3} M atropine (or 2 mg. atropine sulphate, H_2O/ml.), or $5{\cdot}0 \times 10^{-4}$ M oxyphenonium (or 200 μg. oxyphenonium bromide/ml.).
9. 5×10^{-2} M hexamethonium (20 mg. hexamethonium bromide/ml.).
10. $3{\cdot}0 \times 10^{-3}$ M ergotoxine (or 2 mg. ergotoxine ethane sulphonate/ml.).
11. $3{\cdot}5 \times 10^{-3}$ M propranolol (1 mg. propranolol hydrochloride/ml.).
12. $2{\cdot}5 \times 10^{-5}$ M histamine (6 μg. histamine dihydrogen phosphate/ml.).
13. Posterior pituitary extract (vasopressin) 0·5 units/ml.

If a cat is used, both the doses and the stock solutions should be increased 10-fold.

Equipment required:

1. A kymograph and Condon mercury manometer or a blood-pressure transducer, amplifier and recorder.
2. A heated rat operating table with holders and retractors.
3. An overhead lamp.
4. Surgical instruments (p. 7).
5. A tracheal cannula (p. 14).
6. A feather.
7. An arterial cannula made from 1·5 mm. plastic tubing drawn out to about 0·5 mm.
8. A venous cannula as for 7, but the tip may need to be a little less than 0·5 mm.
9. Sutures: 5/0, 3/0 and 1.
10. An injection block (p. 15).
11. A respiration pump may be needed.

Pithed rat as for the anaesthetized rat plus a pithing rod, 2 mm. diameter and about 25 cm. long.

Anaesthetized cat. Items 3 to 8, 13 to 15 and 17 of Experiment 2 (p. 48).

Notes. The rat is a comparatively small animal and is more sensitive to environmental changes than are larger animals. For a steady blood-pressure record to be obtained it is important that the external temperature of the room is kept constant at about 25 to 30°C. or that the animal is kept warm with a heated operating table and overhead lamp. Sudden external changes in temperature are likely to cause variations in blood pressure.

Noradrenaline is more active than adrenaline in causing a rise in blood pressure and isoprenaline will only cause a fall although the increased heart beat may produce an initial rise. After atropine large doses of acetylcholine are required in order to demonstrate the nicotinic effects by producing a rise in blood pressure.

The ergotoxine reversal which was described by Dale[1] can be demonstrated with a number of α-adrenergic blocking agents. The fall in blood pressure caused by adrenaline after α-adrenergic blocking agents can be blocked with propranolol.

This experiment can be modified in many ways, for instance, it can conveniently be used to show the effects of drugs such as propionylcholine (25 nanomoles or 5 μg. propionylcholine iodide), butyrylcholine (250 nanomoles or 50 μg. butyrylcholine iodide), acetyl-β-methylcholine (2·5 nanomoles or 0·5 μg. acetyl-β-methylcholine bromide), carbachol (5 nanomoles or 1 μg. carbachol chloride), and of ephedrine (5 μmoles or 1 mg. ephedrine hydrochloride), amphetamine (2 μmoles or 0·4 mg. amphetamine sulphate) and tyramine (2 μmoles or 0·4 mg. tyramine hydrochloride).

The pithed rat preparation can also be used for a sensitive biological assay of catecholamines. Its sensitivities to adrenaline and noradrenaline are about equal. This enables it to be used in parallel with another preparation, such as the rat uterus (see *Pharmacological Experiments on Isolated Preparations*) in a differential assay procedure

[1] Dale, H. H. (1906). *J. Physiol.*, **34**, 163.

for mixtures of the two amines. A sensitive preparation will respond to about 5 picomoles (1 ng.) of catecholamine, and 250 picomoles (50 ng.) usually give a good response. The samples should be injected on a strict time cycle in volumes not greater than 0·2 ml., washed in with 0·2 ml. saline.

Resistance of the Vascular Bed of the Hind Limb (Fig. 39)

A cat anaesthetized with pentobarbitone (p. 20) is used. The trachea, an external jugular vein and a carotid artery are cannulated and the artery is connected to a mercury manometer or pressure transducer.

The proximal 3 cm. of the femoral artery and femoral vein are dissected free. The femoral nerve is cut. The sciatic nerve is exposed (p. 40) and is also cut. When the dissection is complete, but before cannulation, inject heparin 2,000 i.u./kg. intravenously. Cannulae are inserted into the femoral artery both towards and away from the heart, and are connected by a loop of silicone rubber tubing primed with 0·9 per cent sodium chloride solution. The tubing is passed through a suitable perfusion pump, such as a Watson-Marlow MHRE. Two T-pieces should be connected to the tubing, one on each side of the pump. The downstream T-piece is connected to a mercury manometer or pressure transducer while the upstream T-piece is connected to a three-way tap for close-arterial injection of drugs. The speed of the perfusion pump is adjusted so that the pressure in the perfused femoral artery is equal to that in the cannulated carotid artery. In order to prevent collateral blood flow between the perfused limb and the abdominal circulation, the muscles of the upper thigh can be transected with surgical diathermy. For most purposes, however, it is adequate to tie a tape around the upper thigh excluding the femoral vessels. As flow through the perfused limb is constant, the perfusion pressure can be taken as a measure of vascular resistance.

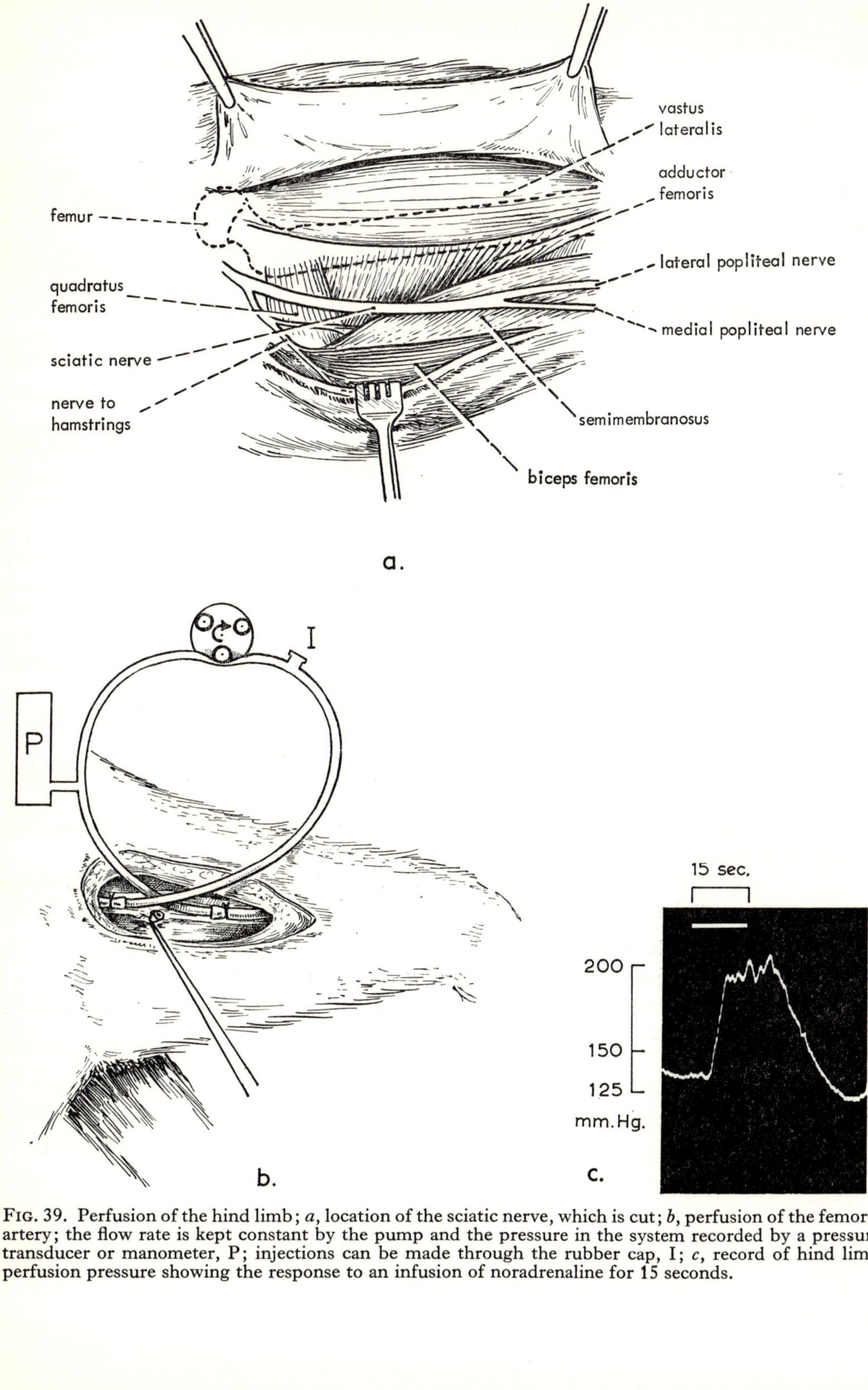

FIG. 39. Perfusion of the hind limb; *a*, location of the sciatic nerve, which is cut; *b*, perfusion of the femoral artery; the flow rate is kept constant by the pump and the pressure in the system recorded by a pressure transducer or manometer, P; injections can be made through the rubber cap, I; *c*, record of hind limb perfusion pressure showing the response to an infusion of noradrenaline for 15 seconds.

Experiment 6: Actions of drugs on vascular resistance. Obtain a pressure/flow curve for the perfused limb by varying the speed of the perfusion pump and recording the perfusion pressure at each speed. Suitable speeds are likely to be between 1 and 20 ml./min.

Return the pump to a speed at which the perfusion pressure equals the cat's systemic arterial pressure, and set up a continuous infusion of adrenaline into the external jugular vein, e.g. by connecting the cannula to an infusion pump or to a burette with a constant head device. The rate of infusion should be about 30 nanomoles (or 10 μg. adrenaline hydrogen tartrate) per minute, so if the volume infused is 0·5 ml./min., the concentration of adrenaline should be 6×10^{-5} M (or 20 μg. adrenaline hydrogen tartrate/ml.). It takes a minute or two after the infusion has started for the pressure to stabilise. When it has, obtain a new pressure/flow curve as quickly as possible; only a few points on the curve can be obtained because tachyphylaxis develops quickly, i.e. the sensitivity decreases.

Repeat the experiment with a similar infusion of noradrenaline. Now return the pump to a speed at which the perfusion pressure equals the cat's systemic arterial pressure. Investigate the effect on perfusion pressure of close-arterial injections into the perfusion circuit of the following drugs:

1. (−)-Noradrenaline, 30 nanomoles (or 10 μg. noradrenaline hydrogen tartrate).
2. (−)-Adrenaline, 30 nanomoles (or 10 μg. adrenaline hydrogen tartrate).
3. (±)-Isoprenaline, 20 nanomoles (or 5 μg. isoprenaline sulphate, B_2, H_2SO_4).
4. Acetylcholine, 50 nanomoles (or 10 μg. acetylcholine idoide).
5. Give phenoxybenzamine, 667 nanomoles (or 200 μg. phenoxybenzamine hydrochloride), and repeat 1, 2 and 3.
6. Give propranolol, 300 nanomoles (or 100 μg. propranolol hydrochloride) and repeat 1, 2 and 3.
7. Give atropine sulphate, 5 nanomoles (2 μg, atropine sulphate, B_2, H_2SO_4, H_2O), and repeat 4.

The blood vessels of the hind limb supply mainly muscle and skin. If the limb is skinned (this must be done before heparin is given), actions of drugs on muscle blood vessels alone are seen. Conversely, the blood vessels of the skin can be studied by perfusing only the paw.

Solutions required:

1. (−)-Noradrenaline, 3×10^{-4} M and 6×10^{-5} M (or 100 and 20 μg. (−)-noradrenaline hydrogen tartrate/ml.).
2. (−)-Adrenaline, 3×10^{-4} M and 6×10^{-5} M (or 100 and 20 μg. (−)-adrenaline hydrogen tartrate/ml.).
3. (±)-Isoprenaline, 2×10^{-4} M (or 50 μg. (±)-isoprenaline sulphate, B_2, H_2SO_4/ml.).
4. Acetylcholine, 5×10^{-4} M (or 100 μg. acetylcholine iodide/ml.).
5. Phenoxybenzamine $3{\cdot}3 \times 10^{-3}$ M (or 1 mg./ml. phenoxybenzamine hydrochloride/ml.).
6. (±)-Propranolol, 3×10^{-3} M (or 1 mg. propranolol hydrochloride/ml.).
7. Atropine sulphate, 5×10^{-5} M (or 20 μg. atropine sulphate, B_2, H_2SO_4, H_2O/ml.).

Equipment required:

1. A perfusion pump such as the Watson-Marlow MHRE fitted with silicone rubber tubing $\frac{1}{16}$ to $\frac{1}{8}$ inch bore according to the size of the animal.
2. A kymograph and two mercury manometers or an electrical recorder and two pressure transducers.
3. A heated operating table.
4. Tracheal, venous and arterial cannulae.
5. Measuring cylinders and a stop watch for calibration of the perfusion pump.

Time required: 6 to 8 hours.

Notes. In the first part of the experiment the drugs are infused intravenously so that their concentrations in the hind limb circulation are independent of blood flow. In the second part of the experiment, since flow is constant, drugs can be given close-arterially, enabling smaller doses to be used. While the demonstration of a changed pressure/flow curve during the infusion of a drug is more instructive and unequivocal than the effect of a single injection, it cannot be achieved with drugs that rapidly induce tachyphylaxis, for which close-arterial injection at constant flow is preferable.

Methods for Studying the Actions of Drugs on the Heart in the Whole Animal

The rate and rhythm of the heart can be studied by electrocardiography with superficial electrodes. This provides a demonstration of one aspect of the effects of a number of drugs on the heart, and is also the basis of a method for a biological assay, of the 'end point' type, of digitalis glycosides.

In order to demonstrate the actions of drugs on the contractility of the heart it is necessary on the one hand to control and measure the venous filling pressure of one or both ventricles, and on the other to compute the external work done by the ventricle in each stroke.

The filling pressure of the ventricles can most easily be measured, with the chest opened by a sternum-splitting incision, by direct cannulation of one or both auricular appendages. A sensitive pressure transducer or a water manometer is required. Filling pressure can be controlled by the method of Sarnoff and Berglund[1] whereby ventricular function curves are obtained by withdrawal of blood followed by stepwise re-injection.

The computation of stroke work ideally involves the continuous recording of flow and pressure of blood at the origin of the aorta or pulmonary artery. This can be done by encircling the vessel with an electromagnetic flow probe, or by diverting its flow through a rotameter. Alternatively, intermittent measurements of cardiac output can be made by a dilution method. If no method for the recording of cardiac output is available it is possible to look at changes in cardiac function by using the correlation found between stroke work and the rate of rise of pressure (dp/dt) in the isometric phase of ventricular contraction.

Changes in contractility induced by drugs can be demonstrated by plotting the relationship between filling pressure and stroke work or dp/dt before, during and after an intravenous infusion of the drug.

Experimental details are not given here, as it is assumed that the setting up of these experiments are beyond the scope of the average student, and will be carried out by demonstrators familiar with the equipment available.

[1] Sarnoff, S. J. & Berglund, E. (1954). *Circulation*, **9**, 706–718.

Recording the Electrocardiogram

The electrocardiogram may be recorded simply by attaching leads to the animal but because the signal from a rat is small it is important that the leads should make good contact and be attached at suitable places. With the anaesthetized rat already set up as described on page 63, it is possible to use needle electrodes inserted through the skin into muscle. If these are arranged as in Figure 40, good records of the electrocardiogram should be obtained. With this preparation it is possible to show the effects of drugs not only on the blood pressure and heart rate but also on the heart muscle itself. It can therefore be used for studying the effects of drugs on arrhythmias and on the conduction of impulses between atria and ventricles.

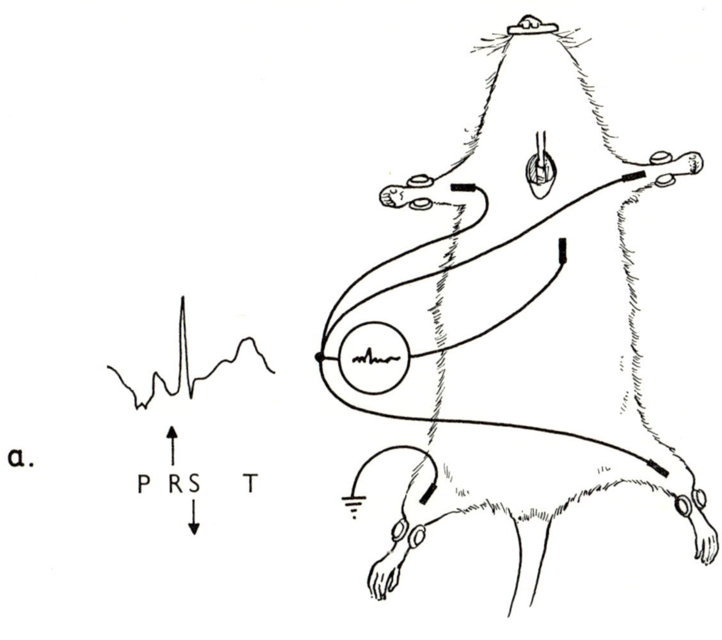

FIG. 40. Recording the electrocardiogram; *a*, typical trace; *b*, suitable positions for electrodes.

Experiment 7: Effects of drugs on cardiac rate and rhythm. Set up the preparation as described above to record blood pressure and the electrocardiogram, with a vein cannulated for the injection of drugs.

1. (–)-Adrenaline. Start with a dose of 5 nanomoles (1 μg. (–)-adrenaline hydrogen tartrate)/kg. and give increasing doses, allowing intervals of 4 to 5 minutes, until a marked but transient effect is seen.
2. Acetylcholine. Proceed as with adrenaline, starting with a dose of 50 nanomoles (10 μg. acetylcholine bromide)/kg.
3. Allow the animal to rebreathe from an anaesthetic bag initially containing about 250 ml. of oxygen until there is a definite increase in respiration. Give doses of acetylcholine and adrenaline that previously failed to induce arrhythmias to demonstrate the potentiation of their actions by respiratory acidosis.
4. Ouabain. Give 400 nanomoles (or 250 μg.) every $2\frac{1}{2}$ minutes until an effect is seen (up to about 6·4 μmoles or 4 mg.). Reverse the effect by giving 10 μmole (or 1 mg.) of potassium chloride every other minute until the normal rhythm is restored.

Solutions required:

1. (–)-Adrenaline, 5×10^{-5} M (or 10 μg. adrenaline hydrogen tartrate/ml.).
2. Acetylcholine, 5×10^{-4} M (or 100 μg. acetylcholine bromide/ml.).
3. Ouabain, 10^{-3} M (or 1 mg./ml.).

Equipment required:

1. Equipment as for rat blood pressure experiment.
2. Low frequency AC amplifier with leads and electrodes for electrocardiography.
3. Pen or optical recorder which will respond rapidly enough so that up to frequencies of 20 Hz the amplitude of the record is not affected by the frequency, i.e. the inertia of the writing system is low.

Time required: 3 to 4 hours.

Notes. This experiment should illustrate some of the points raised in the introduction to this section.

Human Circulation

It is possible to study the effects of drugs on the circulation in man with quite simple apparatus. The pulse rate can be measured adequately by counting the number of beats over a period of 30 seconds; the radial artery is convenient to use for this purpose. The blood pressure can be measured with a sphygmomanometer and stethoscope. The cuff is inflated and the pressure slowly released until the sounds in the stethoscope indicate that the blood is entering the artery intermittently. The pressure at which this occurs indicates the systolic blood pressure. When the cuff is deflated further it should be possible to detect the point at which it does not interfere with the flow of blood through the artery even during diastole. The pressure at which this occurs indicates the diastolic blood-pressure.

In an experiment to test the action of drugs it is important that the subject should be disturbed as little as possible; it is best to use a couch or at least a comfortable chair. It is also important to allow time for the blood pressure and heart rate to become settled before the injection of the drug. Control readings should be taken every five minutes and should clearly be seen to be steady before proceeding. Because most subjects have a certain (natural) apprehension about the experiment, these readings are likely to be abnormal. It is advisable to arrange that some subjects receive a blank injection of sterile saline and that they know of this possibility but do not know whether they are receiving the blank or the drug.

The problem with using human circulation to test the effect of drugs is to assess the safety of the experiment. Risks which may have to be taken in clinical research on new drugs are not acceptable for teaching purposes, particularly with the limited staff and facilities usually available in academic departments of pharmacology. The difference between the dose of atropine which produces effects in man and the toxic dose, however, is very great indeed, and the following experiment has been in use in this department for over twenty years.

Experiment 8: Effects of atropine on man.

Record: 1. The pulse rate, see above.
2. Systolic and diastolic blood pressure, see above.
3. Pupil diameter, the near point, and the briskness of the light reflex (p. 60).
4. The salivary index.
5. The rate of respiration.
6. Any subjective phenomena (sensations of heat, cold, dryness or drowsiness).

To test the salivary index the subject swallows repeatedly so as to remove any saliva from the mouth. Four drops of lemon juice are placed on his tongue and allowed to act for 30 sec. The mouth is rinsed for 15 sec. with 5 ml. of water (conveniently measured with a disposable syringe) and the subject then spits the contents of his mouth into a funnel placed in a measuring cylinder. He continues to empty the contents of his mouth by spitting into the funnel for a further 15 sec. The froth on the collected washings is broken by touching it with a glass rod dipped in octyl alcohol and the volume of the rinsings is noted. By subtracting 5 ml. from this, the volume of saliva, secreted in response to the stimulus of the lemon juice, is obtained and this is recorded as the 'salivary index'. It is worth recording the subject's own assessment of his salivary secretion ('profuse', 'moderate', 'scant', 'nil') and comparing this with the observer's assessment from the appearance of the tongue as well as with the actual volume secreted.

The rate of respiration should be measured over a period of 1 min. if possible without the subject being aware that his respirations are being counted.

Measurements are recorded every 5 min. except those on salivation which are recorded every 10 min. At least two observers are required for each subject. It is better to have three to ensure that records are properly kept and also that the subject is not tempted to help by making some of the measurements himself.

When the control values are steady, the subject is given a subcutaneous injection in the outer aspect of the upper arm with full antiseptic precautions. The skin is swabbed with an antiseptic such as chlorhexidine B.P. and sterile (disposable) syringes and needles are used. The solutions for injection are either atropine sulphate, 2 mg./ml. ($5{\cdot}8 \times 10^{-3}$ M), or sterile saline, and are identified by a suitable code letter. The dose is 0·02 mg. atropine sulphate/kg. body weight (i.e. 58 nanomoles/kg.) so a subject weighing 70 kg. would receive 0·7 ml. of either the atropine sulphate solution or of sterile saline. Some subjects can definitely be given atropine and so serve as controls, but there is usually no difficulty in deciding which subjects have had atropine. Readings are continued after the injection at the same intervals as before and only stopped when it is clear either that the subject received no atropine or that the effects of the atropine have worn off.

Equipment required:

For each subject:

1. Watch with second hand.
2. Stethoscope.
3. Sphygmomanometer.
4. Couch.
5. Pupilometer.
6. Small type chart and ruler.
7. Torch.
8. Lemon juice.
9. Filter funnel.
10. 25 ml. measuring cylinder.
11. Octyl alcohol.
12. Sterile disposable syringes (1 ml. and 5 ml.) and needles.
13. Chlorhexidine solution and cottonwool.
14. Ampoules containing 1 ml. sterile solution of either atropine sulphate (2 mg./ml.) or sterile saline.

Time required: about 2 hours.

Notes. This experiment should show clearly the effects of atropine on salivation and heart rate. It should be noted that the effects on the eye are very slight compared with those when atropine is applied direct to the eye. Contrast the results with those of the much less potent homatropine, observed in Experiment 4, p. 60. It will be seen that in spite of the change in pulse rate, the effects on blood pressure are small and variable. Effects on the respiration are sometimes observed but it is important to note the control results with the saline injection before attaching too great a significance to the small effects. The subject's experience of dryness is very striking and it may be accompanied by warmth and drowsiness, though again this is often observed with the controls once the injection is over, particularly if the experiment is performed in a warm room after lunch.

CHAPTER IV

RESPIRATORY ACTIONS OF DRUGS

Methods for Recording Respiration

1. Gaddum's respirometer (Fig. 41). The animal breathes through a slight constriction, thus causing a fall in pressure in the system when it breathes in. The fall in pressure is recorded by a lever mounted on a tambour and so produces a downward line on a smoked paper. It is calibrated at the end of the experiment by replacing the animal by an aspirator. When water is allowed to flow out of the aspirator, air enters the system at the same rate. The rate of flow of the water is measured with a measuring cylinder and a watch with a second hand and the depression of the lever corresponding to various rates of flow can thus be recorded. This method can be useful for recording respiratory rate, but the amplitude of the record is only crudely related to the size of a breath.

2. Krogh's spirometer (Fig. 42). Here the animal breathes in and out of a closed system including a light copper float over a water seal. Movements of the float are directly related to movements of air in and out of the animal's chest. The float can be attached to a frontal writing lever or to a low-torque potentiometer for electrical recording. The main disadvantage of this method is that the composition of the air in the closed system tends to change as the animal absorbs oxygen and expires carbon dioxide. The system can be filled with pure oxygen and a canister of soda lime incorporated to remove carbon dioxide. The excursions obtained are proportional to tidal volume except at high respiratory rates when the inertia of the system makes the amplitude dependent on frequency.

3. The pneumotachograph (Fig. 43). If a fine wire gauze is introduced into a stream of air a pressure difference is produced across the gauze. If the flow is laminar (streamlined rather than turbulent), the pressure difference is proportional to the flow of air. This pressure can be applied to a sensitive differential electromanometer; a velocity dependent voltage is obtained. To derive a volume dependent signal the velocity signal must be passed through an electronic integrator.

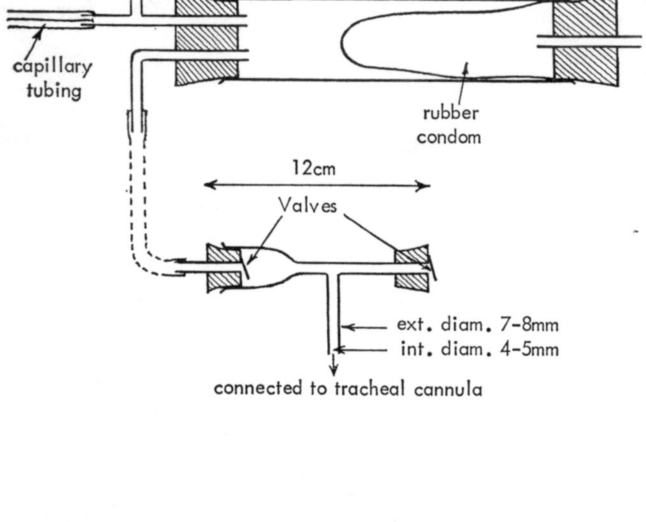

FIG. 41. The Gaddum respirometer. This is attached to the tracheal cannula in the anaesthetized animal. In the original reference (Gaddum, J. H., 1941, *J. Physiol.*, **99**, 257) the apparatus was attached to a mask fitted over the face of a conscious animal.

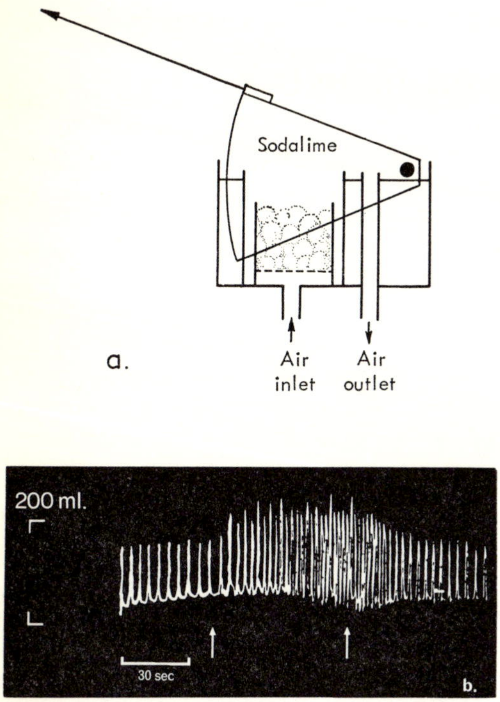

FIG. 42. *a*, The Krogh spirometer; *b*, record obtained with a Krogh spirometer showing increased respiration due to inhalation, between the arrows, of carbon dioxide.

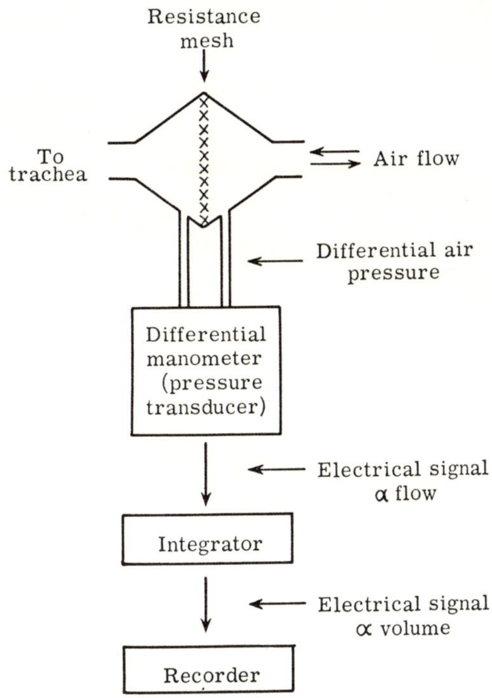

FIG. 43. The pneumotachograph. The difference in pressure between the air on either side of the resistance is recorded by a sensitive manometer.

The Anaesthetized Cat or Rabbit Preparation for Studying the Effects of Drugs on Respiration

Either cats or rabbits may be used. The rabbit is anaesthetized by the injection of urethane (7 ml./kg. of a 25 per cent w/v solution in distilled water) slowly into the marginal vein of the ear (p. 11). Usually 2 to 5 ml. produce anaesthesia and the rest of the dose is given during a period of about 15 minutes; for a rabbit weighing $2\frac{1}{2}$ to 3 kg. the total volume needed may be as much as 20 ml. and the effects usually last for at least five hours. The cat is anaesthetized by the injection of pentobarbitone sodium, 40 mg./kg. i.p. When the animal is relaxed and flaccid, it is secured to the operating table and the fur on the neck removed with electric clippers or cut off with scissors. A tracheal cannula is inserted as described on page 16. The femoral vein or the external jugular vein is cannulated (p. 16) and connected to an injection block which allows a drug to be injected and washed in with saline (Fig. 12). The syringe and cannula are filled with heparinized saline, which is injected in sufficient quantity to fill the unit but too much should not be allowed to enter the animal. A femoral artery is now cannulated and connected to some device for recording the blood pressure (p. 28). The tracheal cannula is connected to a device for the recording of respiration.

Experiment 9 : Drugs and the respiration. Observe the effects on respiration and blood pressure of the following, all drugs being given intravenously:

1. (−)-Adrenaline hydrogen tartrate, 6 to 12 nanomoles; 0·2 to 0·4 ml. of $3{\cdot}0 \times 10^{-5}$ M (10 to 20 μg.).
2. Carbon dioxide introduced into the inspired air; a small pellet of solid carbon dioxide is allowed to vapourize in a 20 ml. plastic syringe and the gas injected through the rubber tubing into the input side of the respirometer.
3. (−)-Morphine hydrochloride $3H_2O$, 10 μmoles; 0·2 ml. of 5×10^{-2} M (4 mg.).
4. Repeat the dose of morphine if the expected effect is not observed. When the respiration is clearly depressed by the morphine, repeat the injection of carbon dioxide into the inspired air (2 above).
5. Nikethamide, 140 to 280 μmoles; 0·2 to 0·4 ml. of 7×10^{-1} M (25 to 50 mg.).
6. When the effect of the nikethamide has worn off, inject (+)-amphetamine sulphate, 5·5 to 16·5 μmoles; 0·1 to 0·3 ml. of $5{\cdot}5 \times 10^{-2}$ M (1 to 3 mg.).
7. When the effect of the (+)-amphetamine has worn off, inject leptazol, 72 μmoles; 0·2 ml. of $3{\cdot}6 \times 10^{-1}$ M (10 mg.).
8. When the effect of the leptazol has passed off, inject nalorphine hydrobromide, 125 to 250 nanomoles; 0·1 to 0·2 ml. of $1{\cdot}25 \times 10^{-3}$ M (0·05 to 0·1 mg.).
9. The respiration should now be about what it was before the injection of morphine; inject thiopentone sodium, 19 μmoles; 0·2 ml. of 10^{-1} M (5 mg.).
10. When the effect of the thiopentone sodium has worn off, inject pentobarbitone sodium, 20 μmoles; 0·2 ml. of 10^{-1} M (5 mg.).
11. Without waiting for the effects of the pentobarbitone to wear off, inject leptazol, 72 μmoles; 0·2 of $3{\cdot}6 \times 10^{-1}$ M (10 mg.).
12. When the stimulant effect of the leptazol has worn off, inject picrotoxin, 1·5 μmoles; 0·1 ml. of $1{\cdot}5 \times 10^{-2}$ M (1 mg.).

Solutions required :

1. (−)-Adrenaline, $3{\cdot}0 \times 10^{-5}$ M (10 μg. (−)-adrenaline hydrogen tartrate/ml.).
2. (−)-Morphine, 5×10^{-2} M (20 mg. morphine hydrochloride, $3H_2O$/ml.).
3. Nikethamide, 7×10^{-1} M (150 mg. nikethamide/ml.).
4. (+)-Amphetamine, $5{\cdot}5 \times 10^{-2}$ M (10 mg. amphetamine sulphate, B_2, H_2SO_4/ml.).
5. Leptazol, $3{\cdot}6 \times 10^{-1}$ M (50 mg. leptazol/ml.).
6. Nalorphine, $1{\cdot}25 \times 10^{-3}$ M (500 μg. nalorphine hydrobromide/ml.).
7. Thiopentone sodium, 10^{-1} M (25 mg. thiopentone sodium/ml.).
8. Picrotoxin, $1{\cdot}5 \times 10^{-2}$ M (10 mg. picrotoxin/ml.).

Equipment required :

1. Equipment as for Experiment 5.
2. Some form of respiratory recording apparatus (see Introduction to this chapter).

Time required : 2 to 3 hours.
Notes. See page 81.

Experiment 10: Sites of action of respiratory stimulants. Prepare the animal as for the previous experiment. Dissect both carotid bifurcations as in the preparation of the superior cervical ganglion (see Fig. 44). Carry out the following tests, both before and after section of both carotid sinus nerves and both vagi in the neck.

1. Change the inspired gas from pure oxygen to oxygen containing 5 per cent carbon dioxide. If a spirometer is used this can be done by allowing the animal to rebreathe oxygen without a soda lime canister.
2. Change the inspired gas from pure oxygen to room air and then to 10 per cent oxygen in nitrogen. If a spirometer is used this can be done by allowing the animal to rebreathe air with a soda lime canister in the system.
3. Intravenous injection of 20 to 60 nanomoles (10 to 30 μg.) of lobeline or 10 to 30 nanomoles (5 to 15 μg.) of nicotine.
4. Intravenous injection of 100 to 200 nanomoles (5 to 10 μg.) of sodium cyanide.
5. Intravenous injection of 140 to 280 μmoles (25 to 50 mg.) of nikethamide.
6. Intravenous injection of 1·5 μmoles (1 mg.) of picrotoxin.
7. Repeat 3, 4 and 5 after an intravenous injection of 3 μmoles (1 mg.) of hexamethonium.

Solutions required:

1. Lobeline, 2×10^{-4} M (100 μg. lobeline hydrochloride/ml.).
2. Nicotine, 10^{-4} M (or 50 μg. (−)-nicotine di(hydrogen tartrate), $2H_2O$/ml.).
3. Sodium cyanide, 2×10^{-3} M (100 μg. sodium cyanide/ml.).
4. Nikethamide, 7×10^{-1} M (50 mg. nikethamide/ml.).
5. Picrotoxin, 10^{-2} M (10 mg. picrotoxin/ml.).
6. Hexamethonium, 3×10^{-2} M (10 mg. hexamethonium bromide/ml.).

Equipment required: As for Experiment 10.

Time required: 5 to 6 hours.

Notes. This experiment separates drugs that act on structures in the brain from those that stimulate chemoreceptors innervated by the ninth and tenth cranial nerves, by a comparison of responses seen before and after denervation of the peripheral receptors. One can only interpret the results qualitatively, as the denervation procedure involves other sensory and motor fibres which modify the quantitative responses to stimulation of central receptors.

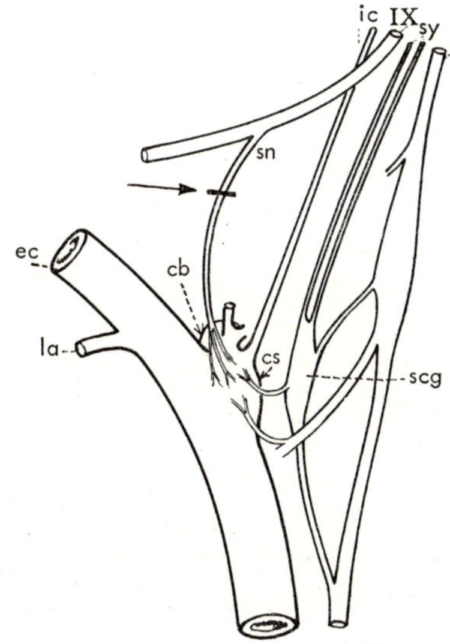

FIG. 44. Location of the carotid body (cb) and carotid sinus (cs); the arrow indicates the point at which the sinus nerve should be cut.

Chapter V

ACTIONS ON THE CENTRAL NERVOUS SYSTEM

The effects of drugs on the central nervous system can be very varied, ranging from alterations in behaviour to depression of the respiration. Drugs which act centrally are extremely important and include many substances which are widely used in medicine. Nevertheless, because their actions are usually complex, it is difficult to design experiments which really show how the effects are brought about. It is also often difficult to assess the effects quantitatively. Although it is relatively simple to observe how long an animal is asleep, it is more difficult to assess the effect of an analgesic and it is usually very difficult indeed to make a quantitative assessment of the effects of a drug on behaviour. Because of the present interest in drugs which affect behaviour a list of doses likely to produce effects is given after the two experiments dealing with analgesia and sleeping time. Details of attempts to assess the effects of drugs on behaviour can be obtained elsewhere[1].

Methods of Assessing Analgesia[2,3]

Most tests for analgesia depend on the application of an external stimulus to an animal and the observation of typical changes in behaviour by which the animal attempts to escape from the situation. In many tests the animal's response is a squeak, in others it moves the part of it which is hurt and in others, in which heat is applied to the feet, it may move its fore-paws and blow on them. In all these tests it is not possible to say that the sensations in the animal are similar to those experienced by man and that the animal feels pain in exactly the same degree as man does. Results obtained in animals, however, may give some guide to the activity of drugs in man, especially if they are potent substances such as morphine or methadone.

[1] Nodine, J. H. & Siegler, P. E. (1964). *Animal and Clinical Pharmacologic Techniques in Drug Evaluation.* Chicago: Year Book Publishers.

[2] Green, A. F. & Young, P. A. (1951). *Br. J. Pharmac.*, **6**, 572.

[3] Millar, R. A. & Stephenson, R. P. (1956). *Br. J. Pharmac.*, **11**, 27.

Many different noxious stimuli, pressure, heat or electric shocks, can be used for testing analgesics and the effects of drugs can be assessed either as graded responses or quantally. To obtain a graded response with a drug it is necessary to be able to measure physically the stimulus giving rise to pain, or rather to the animal's response which is taken to indicate pain. After a dose of an analgesic a bigger stimulus should be needed and the effects of a dose of a drug can be assessed either by the increase in the stimulus required or even simply by the size of the stimulus. Groups of animals are given doses of the drugs and, after a suitable time, the stimulus needed to produce a response is determined for each animal. The average stimulus for the group is then plotted against the log dose and from this it may be possible to compare doses producing comparable effects, i.e. comparable stimuli at which the animals react. One serious disadvantage is that occasionally some animals are so affected by the dose of drug that they cease to respond to stimuli high enough even to cause damage to them. This upsets the calculation of the results, because the stimulus must be regarded as infinite, though it is possible to avoid this by assigning an arbitrary but real number instead, or by using the reciprocal of the stimulus instead of the stimulus itself. Even if the calculation is modified so that results can be obtained they are unlikely to be reliable and, moreover, it is highly undesirable that the animals should be so stressed.

If the responses are assessed quantally, the stimulus is set at a fixed level and each animal is tested to see whether it reacts not or. The probit (Appendix I) of the proportion in each group showing analgesia is then plotted against the log dose and again it may be possible to compare doses producing comparable effects. Usually the standard response is taken as analgesia in 50 per cent of the group of animals and comparisons are made of the dose producing this effect, ED_{50}. It should be remembered that the value of ED_{50} will depend upon the level of stimulus selected. This method has the advantage that it is quicker than finding the threshold stimulus for each animal and moreover it does not give rise to the situation in which infinite values can be obtained and damage done to the animals.

Experiment 11: Comparison of analgesic activity. Pressure can be applied to a rat's tail with the apparatus shown in Figure 45. The plunger of a syringe is placed 1 cm. from the end of the tail and the pressure in the system is raised, by means of a second syringe, until the rat squeaks. By turning a tap the pressure on the tail is released immediately, without releasing the pressure in the manometer, which is recorded. With rats from 3 to 6 weeks old, a pressure of 400 to 500 mm. Hg is usually needed; with older rats it may be necessary to use pressures as high as 600 to 850 mm. Hg.

The test is conducted quantally and the pressure used for testing for the presence of analgesia is usually twice the mean value for untreated animals, i.e. 800 to 1,000 mm. Hg for young rats and 1,200 to 1,700 mm. Hg for older ones. Damage to the rat's tail is only likely to occur with pressures about eight times the threshold value in untreated animals.

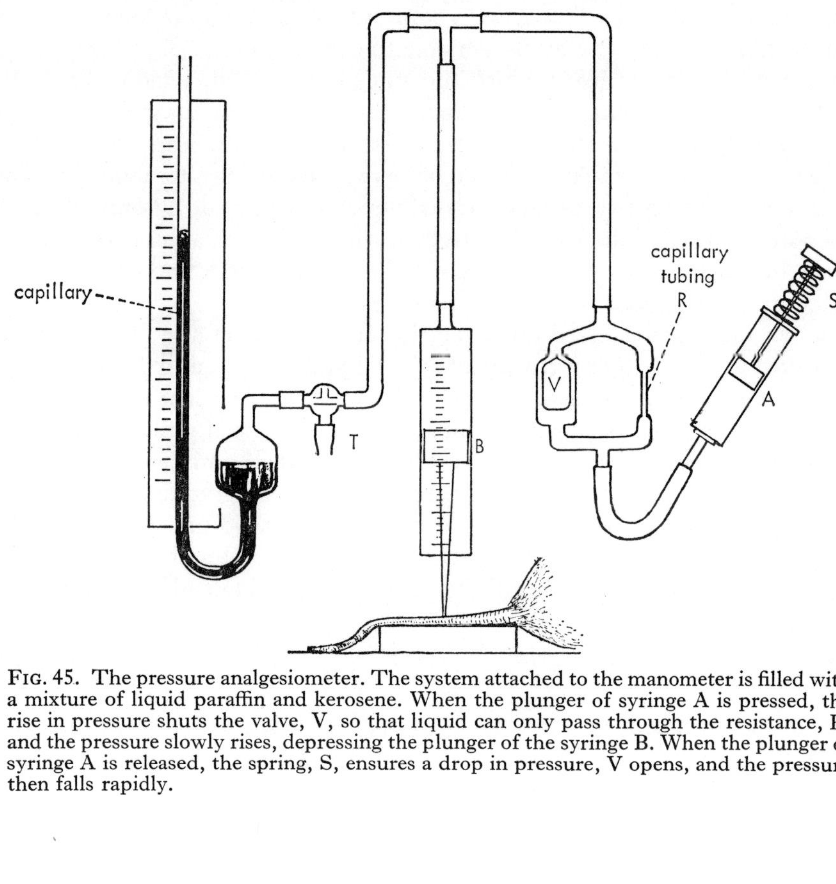

FIG. 45. The pressure analgesiometer. The system attached to the manometer is filled with a mixture of liquid paraffin and kerosene. When the plunger of syringe A is pressed, the rise in pressure shuts the valve, V, so that liquid can only pass through the resistance, R, and the pressure slowly rises, depressing the plunger of the syringe B. When the plunger of syringe A is released, the spring, S, ensures a drop in pressure, V opens, and the pressure then falls rapidly.

For the comparison of two drugs, such as morphine and methadone, the mean threshold pressure is first calculated by measuring the pressure at which the untreated animals respond. They are then divided into eight groups with at least five rats in each group. The drug is given subcutaneously and the following doses are likely to be suitable:

Morphine sulphate, 1·25, 2·5, 5·0 and 10·0 mg./kg. (3·3, 6·6, 13·2 and 26·4 μmoles/kg. i.e. 0·1 ml./100 g. of $3{\cdot}3 \times 10^{-3}$, $6{\cdot}6 \times 10^{-3}$, $1{\cdot}32 \times 10^{-2}$ and $2{\cdot}64 \times 10^{-2}$ M solutions).

Methadone hydrochloride, 0·675, 1·25, 2·5 and 5·0 mg./kg. (2·0, 4·0, 8·0 and 16·0 μmoles/kg., i.e. 0·1 ml./100 g. of $2{\cdot}0 \times 10^{-3}$, $4{\cdot}0 \times 10^{-3}$, $8{\cdot}0 \times 10^{-3}$ and $1{\cdot}6 \times 10^{-2}$ M solutions).

Each rat is tested 30 minutes after the injection with a pressure twice the value of the mean threshold pressure. The number of animals in each group which does not respond to the stimulus is converted into a percentage and the probit corresponding to this obtained from tables. There should be a linear relationship between log dose and the probit of the percentage of animals showing analgesia, and with the doses chosen it is likely that in some groups more than half the animals will show analgesia whereas in others less than half will. It is therefore possible to calculate, either graphically or by algebra, the dose which would produce analgesia in 50 per cent of a group of animals (ED_{50}).

Solutions required:

Morphine sulphate (B_2, H_2SO_4, $5H_2O$), 1·25, 2·5, 5·0 and 10·0 mg./ml., i.e. 3·3, 6·6, 13·2 and $26{\cdot}4 \times 10^{-3}$ M.

Methadone hydrochloride, 0·675, 1·25, 2·5 and 5·0 mg./ml., i.e., 2·0, 4·0, 8·0 and $16{\cdot}0 \times 10^{-3}$ M.

Equipment required:

Apparatus for applying pressure (Fig. 45).
At least eight groups of five rats, 3 to 6 weeks old.
Sterile syringes and needles.

Time required: About 2 hours, if two people are involved.

Notes. The effect is measured 30 minutes after the injection and the experiment must be modified if the time-course of the effects of the drugs are to be compared properly.

Analgesic effects are produced by phenazocine in about one-fifth of the dose of morphine, by phenadoxone in about one-fourth the dose of morphine, by pethidine in about three times the dose of morphine and by codeine in about eight times the dose of morphine.

Sleeping Time in Animals

Many drugs depress the central nervous system and produce unconsciousness or sleep. In animals such as rats and mice the righting reflex can be used to assess whether or not they are 'asleep'. If they are placed on their backs, they normally turn over immediately. If they are given a suitable dose of a drug they can be placed on their backs and the time after the administration of the drug at which they right themselves is taken as the 'sleeping time' and indicates the duration of action of the dose of drug.

Experiment 12 : The duration of action of some barbiturates. Mice are arranged in groups of 5 or 10 animals and the members of each group all receive the same dose of drug/kg. body weight. For the most satisfactory results the drugs should be given intravenously, which necessitates learning the technique of intravenous injections into the tail vein (p. 12). Some success may be obtained with intraperitoneal injections but there are usually some animals which either do not go to sleep at all or which sleep for an infinite period if the drug is given by this route and this makes it impossible to perform quantitative comparisons. It is possible to use experimental results in which some animals have died by taking the reciprocal of the sleeping time for comparison with log dose but a suitable choice of dose and route of administration should avoid the need for this.

Measure the sleeping time in groups of mice which have received the following doses of drugs: Thiopentone sodium, 100, 141 and 200 μmoles/kg. (25, 35·4 and 50 mg./kg.); this is 2, 2.83 and 4 μmoles/20 g. mouse (0·5, 0·71 and 1·0 mg./20 g. mouse) and is contained in 0·1 ml. of 2×10^{-5} M, $2{\cdot}83 \times 10^{-5}$ M and 4×10^{-5} M (5 mg./ml., 7·1 mg./ml. and 10 mg./ml.) solutions. Thialbarbitone sodium, 300, 424 and 600 μmoles/kg. (75, 106 and 150 mg./kg.); this is 6, 8·5 and 12 μmoles/20 g. mouse (1.5, 2.1 and 3.0 mg./20 g. mouse) and is contained in 0·1 ml. of 6×10^{-5} M, $8{\cdot}5 \times 10^{-5}$ M and 12×10^{-5} M (15 mg./ml., 21 mg./ml. and 30 mg./ml.) solutions.

Calculate the mean sleeping time for each group and the standard error and compare the mean values for significance. Select values which are suitable for making a four-point assay, but check that this is justified by comparing the slopes of the two log dose response lines. If it is possible to make an assay, express the potency of thialbarbitone relative to that of thiopentone and calculate the fiducial limits (see Appendix III of the companion volume).

Solutions required :

Thiopentone sodium, 2, 2·83 and 4×10^{-5} M (5, 7·1 and 10 mg. thiopentone sodium/ml.).

Thialbarbitone sodium, 6, 8·5 and 12×10^{-5} M (15, 21 and 30 mg. thialbarbitone sodium/ml.).

Equipment required:

Syringes and needles.

Holder for intravenous injections in mice (Fig. 9).

Dormitory consisting of compartments in which mice can be placed separately when on their backs (this can conveniently be made of cardboard).

Time required: 2 hours or longer, depending on the number of mice used and the skill of the person making the injections.

Notes. For injections by the intraperitoneal route it may be necessary to give up to five times the amounts used intravenously but the results are very variable. Other barbiturates may be used and the following doses are likely to be effective: hexobarbitone sodium, 300 to 600 μmoles/kg. (75 to 150 mg./kg.); pentobarbitone sodium, 120 to 240 μmoles/kg. (30 to 60 mg./kg.); with phenobarbitone sodium the log dose-response curve is very steep and mice tend either to sleep for an infinite period or not at all. The experiment can be modified so as to demonstrate the prolonging of sleeping time produced by chlorpromazine or SKF 525A and the shortening of sleeping time by stimulants such as nikethamide, leptazol and picrotoxin as well as by amphetamines.

Doses of Centrally Acting Drugs effective in Mice

The list shows the range of dose likely to produce detectable effects in mice. It can be used for the qualitative demonstration of the convulsant and anticonvulsant effects of drugs, of the effects of tranquilizers, of the Straub reaction, and so on, but where a quantitative method can be devised for assessing the effect it may be found that smaller doses are needed. The dose of morphine, for example, is about 10 times that used for producing analgesia in rats in Experiment 11.

Oxotremorine, 0·5 to 4·0 μmoles/kg. i.p. (0·1 to 0·8 mg./kg.).

These effects are usually blocked by pretreatment with atropine, 15 μmoles/kg. i.p. (5 mg. atropine sulphate, B_2, H_2SO_4, H_2O/kg.).

Amphetamine, 20 to 40 μmoles/kg. i.p. or 40 to 80 μmoles/kg. orally (amphetamine sulphate, B_2, H_2SO_4, 4 to 8 mg./kg. and 8 to 16 mg./kg. respectively).

Leptazol, 200 to 500 μmoles/kg. i.p. (30 to 90 mg./kg.).

Picrotoxin, 7·5 to 30 μmoles/kg. i.p. (5 to 20 mg./kg.).

Apomorphine, 30 μmoles/kg. i.p. (10 mg. apomorphine HCl, $\frac{1}{2}H_2O$/kg.).

Morphine, 100 to 250 μmoles/kg. i.p. (40 to 100 mg. morphine sulphate, B_2, H_2SO_4, $5H_2O$/kg.).

Phenytoin, 40 to 200 μmoles/kg. i.p. (10 to 50 mg. phenytoin sodium/kg.).

Chlordiazepoxide, 80 to 320 μmoles/kg. i.p. (25 to 100 mg. chlordiazepoxide hydrochloride/kg.).

Meprobamate, 200 μmoles/kg. i.p. (40 mg./kg.).

Chlorpromazine, 30 to 75 μmoles/kg. i.p. (10 to 25 mg. chlorpromazine hydrochloride/kg.); much smaller doses, around 1 μmole (0·3 mg.)/kg. s.c. are likely to prolong the effects of barbiturates on sleeping time.

Reserpine, 16 μmoles/kg. i.p. (10 mg./kg.).

Hexobarbitone, 300 μmoles/kg. i.p. (72 mg. hexobarbitone sodium/kg.).

Chapter VI

ACTIONS ON CERTAIN ORGANS

Many drugs produce their effects by actions on organs associated with special processes, e.g. the liver, kidneys or glands producing hormones. Drugs affecting the kidney are particularly important and their effects can easily be demonstrated in the anaesthetized animal.

The Anaesthetized Cat or Rabbit Preparation for Studying Diuretics[1]

Male animals should be used. Although rabbits are cheaper than cats, there is sometimes considerable trouble in obtaining a satisfactory flow of urine with them, probably because the ureters and bladder are fairly easily damaged. There is usually no trouble when cats are used.

Anaesthesia is produced in rabbits by injecting urethane (7 ml./kg. of a 25 per cent w/v solution in water) slowly into the marginal vein of the ear (p. 11). The trachea is cannulated and then the femoral vein (p. 16). Anaesthesia is induced in cats with halothane (p. 19) and the trachea and the femoral vein cannulated. Anaesthesia is then maintained with chloralose (40 to 80 mg./kg.). Most diuretics produce their effects on the kidneys in doses which do not affect the blood pressure so there is usually little point in recording it and the animal need not be given heparin.

To induce a flow of urine the venous cannula is connected to a 50 ml. burette, fitted with a constant pressure device and screw clip (*Companion volume* Fig. 29), containing 4 per cent dextrose and 0·22 per cent sodium chloride. The head of pressure should be adjusted to give a flow of about 1 ml./min. At least 30 minutes are allowed to elapse after the start of the infusion before any drugs are given.

To collect the urine it is necessary to insert a catheter into the bladder. Suitable catheters can be made of rubber (No. 10 (French gauge) for a cat and No. 8 (French gauge) for a rabbit) or from suitable Portex vinyl tubing. These should have a hole in the side of the tube 5 to 10 mm. from the tip, to reduce the risk of blockage. The catheter is lubricated with glycerol or liquid paraffin. The penis is held with the thumb and forefinger of one hand and the tip of the catheter gently inserted with the other. It is gently pushed in at the same time as being twisted clockwise and anti-clockwise. Its position may be felt by palpating the abdomen but the real test of whether it is in the bladder or not is whether urine flows through it. When it is in place the tube should be fixed in position with adhesive tape. The urine flowing through the catheter is collected in a

[1] Burn, J. H. (1952). *Practical Pharmacology*, p. 53. Oxford: Blackwell.

graduated measure. The first sample may contain blood, caused by damage during the insertion of the catheter, and should be discarded. Subsequent samples are tested for their pH, sodium, potassium and chloride ion content, and from this information and the rate of production of urine is it possible to calculate the rates of excretion of sodium, potassium and chloride ions.

The pH of the urine can be measured with a pH meter or with indicator paper.

The sodium and potassium ion concentrations can be measured with a flame photometer. The instrument is calibrated by using solutions of known concentration, usually in the range $0{\cdot}5$ to $3{\cdot}0 \times 10^{-4}$ M. The urine samples require dilution before the concentrations can be estimated, usually 200-fold for potassium and 750-fold for sodium.

The chloride ion concentration is estimated by adding excess silver nitrate and back-titrating with standard ammonium thiocyanate (Volhard's method). If a 1·0 ml. sample of urine is taken, it is likely that 1·0 ml. of $7{\cdot}5 \times 10^{-2}$ M silver nitrate will provide an excess. The silver nitrate solution should contain nitric acid and a ferric salt which acts as indicator for the back-titration with ammonium thiocyanate. The actual content per litre is 12·75 g. silver nitrate, 250 ml. concentrated nitric acid and 250 ml. of a saturated aqueous solution of ferric ammonium sulphate; 1·0 ml. of this solution is equivalent to 75 μequivalents of chloride. The ammonium thiocyanate should be $3{\cdot}75 \times 10^{-2}$ M, i.e. 2·0 ml. will be equivalent to 1·0 ml. of the silver nitrate reagent.

Experiment 13: The effects of some diuretics. Urine is collected from an animal prepared as described above and tested for its pH, sodium, potassium and chloride ion content. It is usually necessary to collect samples during a period of 10 minutes (or longer if the rate of flow is slow) and a number of control samples should be taken to test that the rate of flow and the composition of the urine are reasonably constant before the drugs are tested.

Investigate the effects of intravenous administration of injection of mersalyl B.P. (0·1 ml. for a rabbit, 0·2 ml. for a cat; these doses contain 10 mg. and 20 mg. respectively of the sodium salt of mersalyl acid, i.e. 20 and 40 μmoles, together with rather less than an equivalent amount of theophylline). After two samples have been collected, i.e. about 20 minutes, injection of dimercaprol B.P. (0·2 ml. for a rabbit, 0·4 ml. for a cat; these doses contain 10 and 20 mg. respectively, approximately 100 and 200 μmoles) is given intramuscularly. Two further samples are collected and tested.

Acetazolamide (30 to 100 mg. for a rabbit; 60 to 200 mg. for a cat; 130 to 500 μmoles and 260 to 1,000 μmoles respectively) is now injected intravenously and further samples are collected. If the expected effect is not observed, the acetazolamide may be added to the intravenous infusion of dextrose and saline in such a concentration that the animal receives about 50 mg. acetazolamide/hr.

Solutions required:

0·9 per cent sodium chloride.
Injection of mersalyl B.P.
Injection of dimercaprol B.P.
Acetazolamide, 1·0 M (250 mg. acetazolamide sodium/ml.).
Standard sodium and potassium solutions for calibration of the flame photometer, in the range 0·5 to $3{\cdot}0 \times 10^{-4}$ M.
Silver nitrate, $7{\cdot}5 \times 10^{-2}$ M, containing nitric acid and a ferric salt (p. 89).
Ammonium thiocyanate, $3{\cdot}75 \times 10^{-2}$ M.

Equipment required:

Equipment for anaesthesia.
Venous cannula and apparatus for infusion of saline.
Catheter.
10 ml. measures for collection of urine.
Flame photometer.
pH meter or indicator papers.
Pipettes and burettes for titration of chloride.

Time required: 2 to 3 hours, provided there are enough people for estimations of sodium, potassium and chloride to be made during the performance of the experiment. This requires at least four people, and more if they are not expert.

Notes. The flow of urine produced by mersalyl is stopped by the administration of dimercaprol, which forms a complex with compounds containing mercury and some other metals (but not lead). It should be seen that the excretion of urine is accompanied by excretion of electrolytes. The effect of acetazolamide on urine flow is often rather weak in this experiment but the change in pH is very striking.

Actions on the Thyroid Gland

The thyroid gland is responsible for the production of thyroxine and tri-iodothyronine, which are formed in the gland from inorganic iodide, removed from the blood. The thyroxine and tri-iodothyronine are stored as thyroglobulin but are released as the free amino-acids, the amount released depending on the levels in the blood and being under the control of thyrotrophin, released from the anterior pituitary. Drugs can affect the levels of thyroxine and tri-iodothyronine in the blood by interfering with the uptake of iodide, with the conversion of iodide to thyroxine and tri-iodothyronine, and with the release of these from the stores.

The uptake of iodide by the thyroid gland and the effects of drugs on this uptake can conveniently be studied by injecting an inorganic iodide containing a radioactive isotope of iodine and following the appearance of radioactivity in the thyroid. The most convenient isotope to use is I^{131}, which has a half-life of 8 days and emits both β and γ-radiation. Some other tissue, such as the liver, should be used as a control to demonstrate that the uptake is peculiar to the thyroid and a further check is obtained by measuring the radioactivity in the urine.

Experiment 14: The effects of drugs on the uptake of iodide by the thyroid gland. Six rats, or groups of rats, are treated as follows:

1. Controls, which receive only the dose of labelled iodide.
2. Animals treated with potassium perchlorate (10 mg.), 72 μmoles, injected intraperitoneally 5 minutes *before* the injection of labelled iodide.
3. Animals treated with potassium iodide, (10 mg.), 60 μmoles, injected intraperitoneally 5 minutes *before* the injection of labelled iodide.
4. Animals treated with carbimazole (1 mg.), 5·4 μmoles, injected subcutaneously 1 hour *before* the injection of labelled iodide.
5. Animals treated with carbimazole, as in group 4, and subsequently treated, 3 hours *after* the injection of labelled iodide, with potassium perchlorate (10 mg.), 72 μmoles, injected intraperitoneally.
6. Animals treated with the dose of labelled iodide and *after* 3 hours with potassium perchlorate (10 mg.), 72 μmoles, injected intraperitoneally.

The concentration of labelled iodide is arranged so that it contains 2 microcuries/ml. and each animal receives 0·25 ml. injected intraperitoneally, i.e. 0·5 microcuries. The actual concentration of iodide is unlikely to be isotonic but this is not important because only a small volume is injected intraperitoneally. The rats are placed in cages which have a mesh floor so that the urine can be collected with a funnel and measuring cylinder (Fig. 46) and are all killed 4 hours after the injection of labelled iodide. A convenient way to do this is to inject urethane (25 per cent), 2·8 M intraperitoneally in a dose of 0·7 ml./100 g.

The thyroid gland (Fig. 47) and the liver are dissected out and the liver is weighed to the nearest 100 mg. The radioactivity in the whole thyroid gland determined by placing it in a test tube in the well of a 'Castle' scintillation counter. In this the radiation emitted by the isotope is detected by the flashes of light which it produces from the scintillating material around it. These flashes are converted into electrical impulses by a photo-electric device and are counted for a suitable period. A count is also taken of the radioactivity in a piece of liver about the same size as the thyroid gland, i.e. about 50 mg., and from this the radioactivity of the whole organ is calculated. All these estimates must be corrected by deducting the background radioactivity, which is obtained by making a count with nothing in the well.

To determine the amount of radioactivity in the urine it is first necessary to wash the mesh floor of the cage with water and to add the washing to the urine already collected, together with any urine found in the bladder, which is sucked out with a syringe. The total volume, usually between 40 and 50 ml. is measured in a graduated cylinder and a 2 ml. portion removed with a syringe or safety-pipette and placed in a test-tube, transferred to the well and counted. The total amount of radioactivity in the urine is then calculated.

Note. All estimates of radioactivity should be corrected by deducting the background radiation count and all the results are expressed as a percentage of the count corresponding to the total dose of radioactivity given to the animal. The latter is obtained by making a count with 0·25ml. of a one-tenth dilution of the solution of sodium iodide used and multiplying this by ten.

Solutions required:

1. Labelled sodium or potassium iodide, 2 microcuries/ml.
2. Potassium perchlorate, 100 mg./ml. ($7{\cdot}2 \times 10^{-1}$ M).
3. Potassium iodide, 100 mg./ml. (6×10^{-1} M).
4. Carbimazole, 10 mg./ml. ($5{\cdot}4 \times 10^{-2}$ M).
5. Urethane, 250 mg./ml. (2·8 M).

Equipment required:

1. Scintillation counter.
2. Metabolism cages and measuring cylinders.
3. Syringes, dissecting instruments.
4. Safety-pipettes.

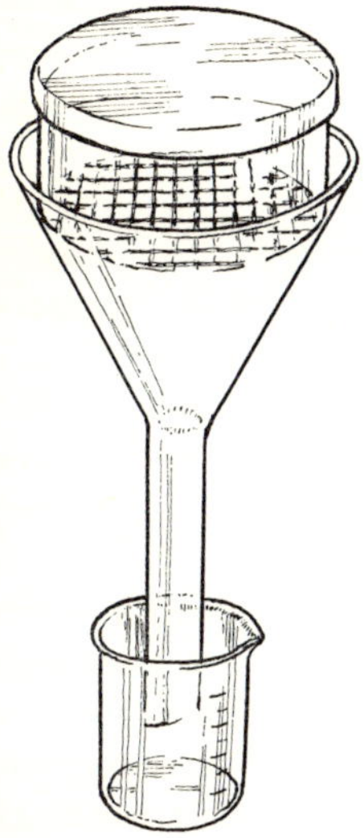

FIG. 46. A simple metabolism cage. The rat is placed on the wire mesh and the urine collects in the beaker.

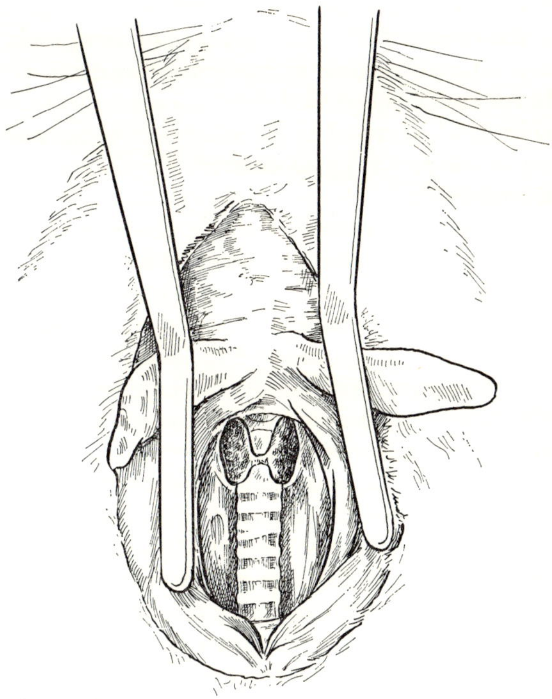

FIG. 47. Location of the thyroid gland in the rat.

Time required: The carbimazole, used in groups 4 and 5, must be given first, the labelled iodide 1 hour later, the rats killed 4 hours after that, and the rest of the experiment takes 2 to 3 hours, i.e. the total time taken is about 8 hours but only the last 2 to 3 involve continuous work.

Notes. The uptake of iodide by the thyroid gland is clearly seen from the animal(s) in group 1. After potassium perchlorate (group 2) or loading the animal with iodide (group 3) there is virtually no uptake of iodide and a high proportion of the radioactivity appears in the urine. After carbimazole (group 4) the uptake of iodide is greatly reduced, though not abolished, but after carbimazole and potassium perchlorate (group 5) there is very little uptake and a high proportion of radioactivity appears in the urine. Potassium perchlorate given 3 hours after the injection of labelled iodide (group 6) has a relatively small effect on the uptake because by this time an appreciable amount of labelled iodide has been incorporated in organic compounds, such as iodotyrosine, from which it is not displaced by the perchlorate anion.

Experiment 15: The effects of drugs on oxygen consumption by rats. The thyroid gland regulates the basal metabolic rate. Indirect information about thyroid function can therefore be obtained by measuring the rate of uptake of oxygen by an animal, which provides a measure of its metabolic rate.

Rats, preferably of uniform weight, are divided into three groups. All rats are pretreated by daily intraperitoneal injections for six days before the measurements are made.

Group I receive carbimazole 5·4 μmoles (1 mg.)/kg. daily.
Group II receive thyroxine 12·9 μmoles (10 mg.)/kg. daily.
Group III receive 0·9 per cent sodium chloride 0·1 ml. daily.

For measurements of oxygen uptake, a rat is placed in the apparatus shown in Figure 48.

The apparatus consists of a chamber for the animal, connected to an air-filled bottle. The bottle has two additional tubes entering it, one from an oxygen cylinder and the other from a 50 ml. burette filled with water. The lower compartment of the animal chamber contains soda lime to absorb the expired carbon dioxide.

The air space of the apparatus is first flushed through with pure oxygen. The connections to the atmosphere are then closed, and a few minutes are allowed for thermal equilibrium to be reached. As the animal takes up oxygen, and its expired carbon dioxide is absorbed by the soda lime, the amount of gas in the apparatus is reduced, and the pressure, recorded by the water manometer, tends to fall. The pressure can be restored to atmospheric pressure by running in water from the burette. If the pressure is adjusted at the beginning and end of a time period, then the volume of water needed represents the volume of oxygen taken up by the animal during the period.

Solutions and reagents required:

1. Carbimazole, $5{\cdot}4 \times 10^{-3}$ M (1 mg./ml.).
2. Thyroxinc, $1{\cdot}29 \times 10^{-2}$ M (10 mg./ml.).
3. Sodium chloride, 0·9 per cent.
4. Granulated soda lime.

Equipment required:

Apparatus as shown in Figure 48.

Notes. For mode of action of carbimazole see notes on previous experiment. These doses of carbimazole and thyroxine have been found to produce approximately a halving and a doubling, respectively, of the metabolic rate.

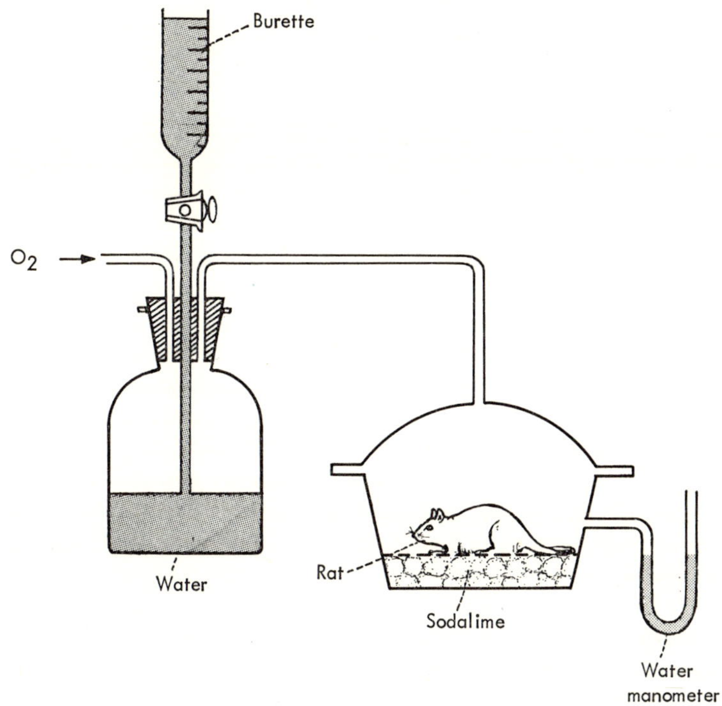

FIG. 48. Apparatus for the measurement of the oxygen consumption of rats.

CHAPTER VII

DRUG EXCRETION AND METABOLISM

In this book we have so far been concerned with the actions of drugs on parts of the body; we now consider the actions of the body upon the drugs themselves. Both what the drug does and what is done to it will determine the overall effect which is observed. How long a drug acts will depend upon how rapidly it is metabolized and/or excreted. How quickly a drug acts largely depends upon how it is given, though this may also affect how long it acts, because it is sometimes possible to place the drug at a site where it is not metabolized and from which it is gradually absorbed.

To study the metabolism and excretion of drugs it is necessary to have methods for estimating them quantitatively. These methods vary from one drug to another but usually involve chemical reactions which produce coloured products, or products which absorb ultraviolet light. The concentration of material which is detected is therefore usually about 10^{-4} M and this is likely to have been obtained by a 50-fold dilution of the original sample, say 0·1 ml. of blood treated to give 5·0 ml. of a material which is coloured or absorbs ultra-violet light. Levels in the blood which can conveniently be measured in this way are therefore around 5×10^{-3} M. Many drugs are active in much lower concentrations than this; some can be detected by fluorescence methods, which are about 10 times as sensitive as methods depending on absorption. Some, such as antibiotics, can be detected by bioassay. With others it may be possible to use tracer techniques. Whatever method is used, it must be established that it is detecting the drug and not metabolites formed from the drug. With a bioassay method it is unlikely that both drug and metabolites will be active and this may also be true in some (but not all) tests involving colour, absorption, or fluorescence. It may well not be true, however, for tests with an isotopically labelled drug in which it is most important to establish, e.g. by chromatography, that the radioactivity comes from the drug and not from a metabolite.

Experiment 16 : Concentrations of sulphacetamide in the blood of rabbits after injection by various routes. Blood samples can conveniently be taken from the marginal vein of the rabbit. The edge of the ear should be shaved or the hair removed by plucking. The animal is given an intravenous injection of heparin (0·5 ml., 1,000 units/kg.); bleeding from the site of the injection is controlled by applying a small piece of cotton wool and a light clip (a light bulldog clip or a domestic hair curler). The animal should be kept warm, particularly the ears which should be gently heated with a lamp for some minutes before any blood sample is taken. It also helps if the edge of the ear is smeared with Vaseline petroleum jelly, so that the blood runs freely over the surface and into the watchglass used to collect the samples. The clip and cotton wool are replaced after the sample has been taken. When the clip is removed and the ear rubbed, bleeding should begin again and samples can easily be taken for the next 2 hours. If the needle used for the injection was very fine it may be necessary to make a slightly larger cut in the vein with a sharp razor or scalpel blade. The animal should be watched to see that it does not remove the clip by scratching. For estimating sulphacetamide samples of 0·2 ml. of blood are adequate, i.e. usually about 10 drops of blood will be enough. The first 2 or 3 drops should be discarded, particularly if the ear has not been kept warm and there is reason to believe that the circulation in the ear has been poor. If the animal has received the sulphacetamide intravenously in one ear vein, it is advisable to take blood samples from the other ear. The drops of blood are collected on a watch-glass and the sample is measured with a blood-pipette fitted with a rubber tube and glass mouth-piece (Fig. 49); the pipette can be held level and the volume adjusted by applying a piece of filter paper to the tip.

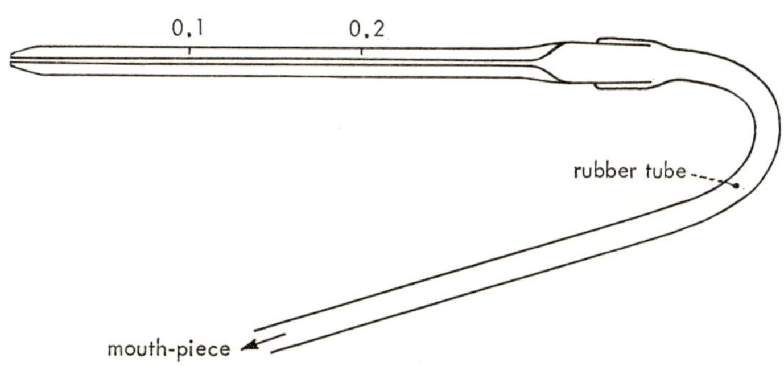

FIG. 49. A blood-pipette, with rubber connection leading to a glass mouth-piece.

The sulphacetamide is estimated, after precipitation of the proteins, by diazotization and coupling with N-(1-naphthyl)ethylenediamine and the purple colour estimated in a colorimeter. The 0·2 ml. sample of blood is added to 3·2 ml. distilled water in a test-tube and the blood-pipette washed by sucking some of the water in and blowing it out again. The blood and water are mixed by shaking them gently and then left for 5 minutes. Trichloracetic acid, 0·6 ml. of a 25 per cent w/v solution, is added and the tube shaken vigorously and left for 5 min. but shaken from time to time. The precipitated proteins are filtered off through a small (e.g. 4·25 cm.) Whatman No. 1 filter paper, with a dry funnel into a dry test tube. Alternatively, the precipitated protein is separated by centrifuging. A volume of 2·0 ml. of filtrate or supernatant is transferred with a pipette to another dry tube. Sodium nitrite, 2 drops of a 0·5 per cent w/v solution, is added, the tube shaken and left for 3 min. Ammonium sulphamate, 1·0 ml. of a 0·5 per cent w/v solution, is added to destroy the excess nitrous acid and the tube left for 2 min, but shaken from time to time. N-(1-naphthyl)ethylenediamine dihydrochloride, 2·0 ml. of a 0·05 percent w/v solution, is added and the tube shaken. After at least 5 min. the colour should be fully developed and the absorption can be measured. The colour does not fade appreciably over a period of an hour.

It is necessary to prepare standard solutions of sulphacetamide in order to obtain the graph of optical density against concentration. These should lie in the range 20 to 200 mg./litre (10^{-4} to 10^{-3} M) and 0·2 ml. samples of these are added to 3·2 ml. distilled water and the trichloracetic acid and other reagents are added as described above, but the filtration can be omitted. The coloured product has an absorption maximum at 500 to 550 mμ and if the optical density is measured with an instrument which uses filters (instead of a monochromator), the one selected should be bright spectrum green, Ilford No. 624. Note that the optical density is directly proportional to the concentration, i.e. the results fit the Lambert-Beer law.

A dose of sulphacetamide sodium, 150 mg./kg. (0·59 mmole/kg.) i.e. 2·0 ml./kg. of a solution containing 75 mg./ml. (approximately 3×10^{-1} M), is administered to five rabbits in different ways; subcutaneously, intramuscularly, intravenously, intraperitoneally and orally. Blood samples are taken before the injection and 10, 30, 60, 90 and 120 min. after the injection. The subcutaneous injection (p. 10) can conveniently be made below the skin on the back and the dose may be divided into two portions. The intramuscular injection (p. 10) is best made deep into the buttock and the dose should be divided into two portions, one into each side of the animal. The intravenous injection (p. 10) must be given slowly and a clip may be necessary to prevent bleeding from the ear, because the animal has received heparin. The intraperitoneal injection is given as described on page 10. The oral administration is sometimes difficult and it may be necessary to inject thiopentone sodium, 2·5 mg./kg. intravenously, to produce anaesthesia and make it easier to pass the stomach tube. The dose of sulphacetamide should be washed in with 50 to 100 ml. of water.

The sample taken before the administration of the drug serves as a blank and is usually quite free from colour. From the calibration curve the concentration in blood is determined and plotted against the time after the drug was given.

Solutions required:

1. Sulphacetamide sodium, 75 mg./ml. (*or* 3×10^{-1} M).
2. Trichloracetic acid, 25 per cent w/v (1·5 M).
3. Sodium nitrite, 0·5 per cent w/v ($7{\cdot}2 \times 10^{-2}$ M).
4. Ammonium sulphamate, 0·5 per cent w/v ($4{\cdot}4 \times 10^{-2}$ M).
5. N-(1-naphthyl)ethylenediamine dihydrochloride, 0·05 per cent w/v ($1{\cdot}9 \times 10^{-3}$ M).
6. Injection of heparin.

Equipment required:

1. Light clips for controlling bleeding.
2. 6 watch-glasses per rabbit for collecting blood samples.
3. 0·2 ml. blood pipettes, one for each animal.
4. Sterile syringes and needles.
5. Razor blades.
6. Vaseline petroleum jelly.
7. Cotton wool.
8. 18 test tubes per rabbit.
9. 5 ml. graduated pipette, 1 ml. graduated pipette, 2×2 ml. and 1×1 ml. bulb pipettes, for each rabbit, plus small funnel and filter paper.
10. Colorimeter or absorptiometer such as a Unicam SP 1300 instrument, with filter No. 624 (Ilford).

Time required: The estimations can be made by one person, though it is often convenient to have two people (i.e. 10 people altogether) and if all five rabbits can be studied simultaneously it takes about $2\frac{1}{2}$ hours from the time the blank samples are taken.

Note. The experiment should show the effect of the way in which the sulphacetamide is given on the initial levels in the blood. An attempt should be made to calculate the maximum level which might be attained and this should be compared with what is observed with the intravenous injection. It should be noted that after an hour the rate of decline in blood level is similar for all methods of administration tested here.

Experiment 17 : Metabolism of ethanol by the rabbit. The concentration of ethanol in blood may be estimated by gas chromatography[1]. A very small amount of ethanol is injected into a stream of nitrogen which passes through a column containing an inert inorganic support, 'Chromosorb', coated with 'Carbowax', a polyethylene glycol preparation. If a substance dissolves in the Carbowax to any extent, it will be held back while substances which do not dissolve are carried along the column by the stream of nitrogen (the 'carrier gas'). As materials emerge from the column they can be detected in a number of ways but one of the most common is with a flame ionization detector. The gas from the column is passed through a flame and organic materials will burn and so produce ions. If electrodes are placed across the flame, these ions will decrease the resistance and a potentiometeric recorder is used to monitor this continuously. The apparatus is shown diagrammatically in Figure 50.

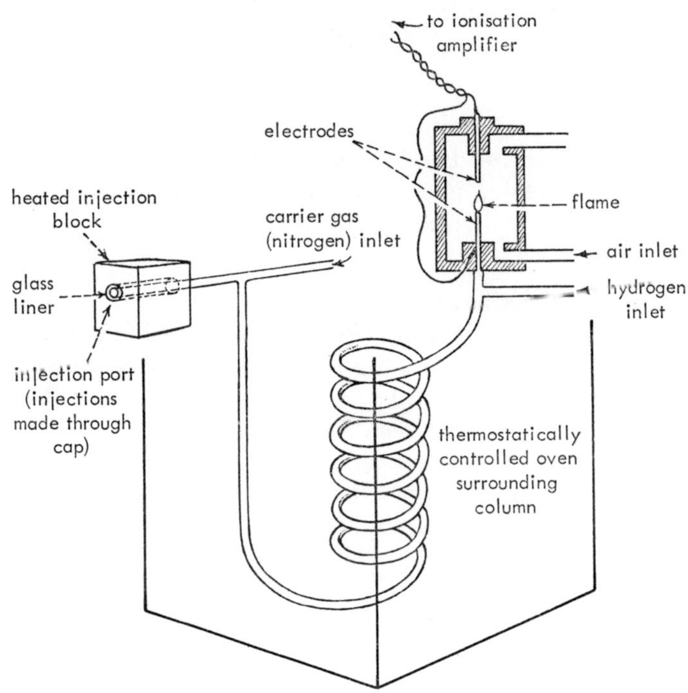

FIG. 50. Gas chromatograph with flame-ionization detector (diagrammatic). The spiral column contains the Chromosorb coated with Carbowax.

[1] Curry, A. S., Walker, G. W. & Simpson, G. S. (1966). *Analyst*, **91**, 742.

The time between the injection of a substance and its appearance in the detector is called the retention time. This varies with temperature because this affects the extent to which the substance dissolves in the Carbowax, and it is essential to keep the column in a thermostatically controlled oven. It is also necessary to heat the injection block so that the material is vapourized when it is inserted into the carrier gas stream. The choice of temperature is determined by the need to vapourize the material and to have a conveniently short retention time but if the column is too hot the retention time may be so short that closely related compounds do not become separated. For this experiment the column temperature should be 70°C.

The amount of material which can be injected without flooding the column depends upon its size but is usually very small, often less than 1 μlitre. Though there is no difficulty in detecting such small quantities, because the electrical detector is extremely sensitive, it is very difficult to measure them with any accuracy, even with specially designed syringes, and it becomes necessary to adopt an internal standard. This is achieved by adding the sample containing ethanol to a solution of propan-1-ol in water (20 mg. per cent, $3{\cdot}3 \times 10^{-3}$ M). At 70° C propan-1-ol has a slightly longer retention time than ethanol, roughly 7 min. as compared with 4 min. using a 2-metre column of Carbowax 400 on Chromosorb W (10:90 w/w). The water does not affect the detector, so when a mixture of ethanol and propanol in water is injected, two clear peaks should be seen. With a Perkin-Elmer F11 instrument a 50-fold attenuation is suitable for the injection of 3 μlitres of the propan-1-ol solution. This usually produces a peak which is between half and three-quarters of the full excursion of the recorder. If 3 μlitres of a mixture of ethanol, propan-1-ol and water is injected on a number of occasions the absolute areas of the peaks will vary, because of the difficulty of injecting exactly the same amount each time, but the relative areas of the two peaks remain constant, because these depend on the relative amounts of ethanol and propan-1-ol. With machines fitted with an integrator these areas can be recorded directly, but if the peaks are very narrow, as should be true if only small amounts are used and the column is achieving good resolution, it is reasonable to use the relative peak heights instead of the areas.

Injections and collection of samples. A rabbit is given an intravenous injection of 5 ml./kg. of ethanol, 20 per cent w/v in normal saline (4·4 M), i.e. it receives 1 g. ethanol/kg. body weight. It also receives 0·2 ml./kg. of heparin, 5,000 units/ml. (i.e. 1,000 units/kg.), as in Experiment 16, and blood samples are taken in exactly the same way as in that experiment but at intervals of 15 minutes (instead of 30 min.) and with 6 or 7 drops of blood because only a 0·1 ml. sample is needed. This is added to 1 ml. of the solution of propan-1-ol in water (20 mg. per cent, $3{\cdot}3 \times 10^{-3}$ M), shaken, and 3 μlitres is injected into the gas chromatograph. The injection port should be fitted with a glass liner to retain blood proteins and prevent them from clogging the column. It is also important to rinse the syringe well between injections. The peak height of the ethanol relative to the peak height for propan-1-ol is compared with the relative heights obtained with injections of known amounts of ethanol and the mixture of propan-1-ol and water.

Tests can be made about once every ten minutes on the gas chromatograph and in addition to making some tests with alcohol solutions of known composition at the start of the experiment, it is advisable also to test them between tests of the samples.

Solutions required:

1. Ethanol 20 per cent w/v (4·4 M) in normal saline.
2. Propan-1-ol 20 mg. per cent w/v ($3{\cdot}3 \times 10^{-3}$ M) in water.
3. Injection of heparin (5,000 units/ml.).

Equipment required:

1. Light clips for controlling bleeding.
2. 16 to 20 watch glasses for blood samples (a smaller number if they are washed and re-used).
3. 0·1 ml. blood pipettes.
4. 1 ml. bulb pipette.
5. Sterile syringes and needles.
6. Razor blades.
7. Vaseline petroleum jelly.
8. Cotton wool.
9. 16 to 20 small tubes (e.g. 2 ml. capacity) with stoppers to prevent evaporation.
10. Gas chromatograph with glass liner in injection block. Microsyringe (e.g. 5 μl. capacity).

Time required: It takes up to an hour to prepare the solutions and to obtain some results with the standard alcohol solutions. It takes from 3 to 4 hours to follow the complete elimination of this dose of alcohol.

Notes. Ethyl alcohol can also be determined by reaction with alcohol dehydrogenase and nicotinamide-adenine-dinucleotide (NAD). The alcohol is converted to acetaldehyde and the NAD reduced to the dihydro- form, NADH, which can be estimated spectrophotometrically. The gas chromatographic method is used here because the technique is widely used for a variety of other compounds as well as being extremely reliable and convenient. It is used in the United Kingdom for the estimation of alcohol in blood samples taken from motorists whose breath gives a positive 'breathalyser' reaction.

The experiment should show that the metabolism of ethanol occurs at virtually a constant rate, independent of the concentration, i.e. it is a zero-order process. At very low concentrations the rate may possibly be slower but it is difficult to be certain of this because this only appears to occur at levels which are near the limit of the sensitivity of the method.

Experiment 18: The influence of acidaemia and alkalaemia on the rate of excretion of aspirin by the kidneys in man. For this experiment students work in pairs, one acting as subject and the other as analyst. The subjects are divided into three groups, of which one is rendered acidotic by the ingestion of ammonium chloride and one is rendered alkalotic by the ingestion of sodium bicarbonate while the third remains in normal acid-base balance. All subjects are given a water load which is maintained throughout the experiment, ensuring that they are able to produce consistent samples of urine at regular intervals. Because of the effects of aspirin on gastric mucosa, students with any history of gastric disorder should not be used as subjects; nor should students who have not previously taken aspirin, because a small proportion of people are abnormally sensitive to its effects.

Procedure:
Time:

0 min. Empty bladder. Take 750 ml. water load.
60 min. Collect urine for volume measurement; drink an equal volume of water.
80 min. Collect urine for volume, pH, and control salicylate estimation. Drink an equal volume of water.
100 min. Collect urine for analysis as above. Take ammonium chloride (130 millimoles, 7 g.), or sodium bicarbonate (120 millimoles, 10 g.) and an appropriate volume of water.
120 min. Collect urine. Drink water. Take aspirin (8·33 millimoles, 1·5 g.).

Collect urine at 20-min. intervals, drinking an equivalent volume of water. Record the volume, pH, and salicylate concentration of each 20-min. sample.

Plot the percentage of the dose of aspirin remaining in the body against time for each of the three groups.

Estimation of Aspirin

Acetyl salicylic acid is hydrolyzed to salicylic acid, which is then estimated colorimetrically. The colour developed with ferric nitrate is standardized using a solution of salicylate of known strength.

To a 50 ml. sample add a few drops of ammonia (S.G. 0·88). Place the sample in a boiling water bath for 10 min., cool, neutralize using indicator paper and make up to 100 ml.

To 1 ml. of water, standard, or hydrolyzed sample add 6 ml. of ferric nitrate reagent. Read the optical density at 525 mμ. The optical density should be proportional to concentration over the range from 0·7 to $3 \cdot 0 \times 10^{-3}$ M, i.e. 100 to 400 μg. salicylic acid per 1 ml. sample. Appropriate dilutions must therefore be made.

Drugs required:

1. Ammonium chloride and sodium bicarbonate either made up in paper sachets in doses of 130 millimoles (7 g.) and 120 millimoles (10 g.) respectively, or dissolved in water and appropriately flavoured.
2. Aspirin tablets 8·33 millimoles (1·5 g.) per subject.

Equipment required:

1 litre measuring cylinders.
pH meter.
Spectrophotometer.

Solutions required

Ferric nitrate reagent, containing ferric nitrate, 9·9 millimoles (4 g. ferric nitrate $9H_2O$), and mercuric chloride, 14·7 millimoles (4 g.) dissolved in N/10 hydrochloric acid (100 ml.). The concentrations of ferric nitrate and mercuric chloride are therefore just below 10^{-1} and $1{\cdot}5 \times 10^{-1}$ M respectively.

Standard salicylate solution, e.g. sodium salicylate, $1{\cdot}25 \times 10^{-3}$ M (200 μg./ml)

Time required: 6 hours.

Notes. If a drug is partially ionized in plasma and urine and is able to diffuse through the walls of the renal tubules only in the non-ionized form, the rate of diffusion will depend on the concentration gradient of the non-ionized form. Any difference in hydrogen ion concentration between urine and plasma will affect the gradient, and therefore the rate of excretion of the drug. Ingestion of acids and alkalis leads to small changes in the hydrogen ion concentration of plasma, which is well buffered, but to large changes in that of urine, while the renal tubules correct the acidaemia and alkalaemia.

Appendix I

THE TREATMENT OF ALL-OR-NONE RESPONSES

When a drug produces an all-or-none response, it is not possible to assess its effect by the intensity of the response produced by a dose. Drugs producing all-or-none responses can only be compared by measuring the doses which produce the effect. Some all-or-none effects are reversible, for example, the blockage of conduction produced by a local anaesthetic acting on a single nerve-fibre. A comparison of two local anaesthetics could therefore be made by comparing the concentrations which just blocked conduction. This would only be valid, however, if the nerve-fibre had recovered fully from the effects of the first drug before the second was tested, i.e. if the sensitivity of the nerve-fibre was the same in the tests with both drugs. Many all-or-none effects, such as death, are not reversible so different drugs must be compared in different animals and it is well known that the sensitivities of different animals are not likely to be the same.

The extent to which sensitivity varies in different animals can be assessed by giving the same drug to a number of them and measuring the amount needed to produce the effect. Experiments were made, for example, in which digitalis was infused at a steady rate into cats until the animals died and the amount of digitalis infused was therefore the lethal dose for each particular animal. In these experiments it was found that the individual lethal doses were scattered more or less symmetrically about a mean value. In experiments with other drugs and animals the extent of the scatter varied but the general shape of the curve was the same, though there is reason to believe that the distribution is more symmetrical if the logarithm of the dose is used instead of the dose itself. The extent of the scatter of individual results about the mean is given by the standard deviation

$$s = \sqrt{\left(\frac{\Sigma d^2}{n-1}\right)}$$

where n is the number of results and d is the deviation of each result (x) from the mean ($\bar{x}$), i.e. $x - \bar{x}$. $\Sigma (x - \bar{x}) = 0$, because $\bar{x}$ is the mean value, but $\Sigma (x - \bar{x})^2$ is positive and is a measure of the scatter of the results from the mean. This is divided by the number of degrees of freedom, $(n-1)$, i.e. the number of pieces of information about the scatter. Although there are n results, there are only $(n-1)$ pieces of information, because with the mean value, $\bar{x}$, and $n-1$ values for x, the nth value can be calculated. If the distribution of individual lethal doses is now considered not in terms of the dose but in terms of the mean dose and the standard deviation, i.e. the dose x is replaced by $\bar{x} \pm Ns$, and N is plotted as the variable, the distribution curves assume a common shape, which is assumed to be that of a normal frequency curve. This expresses purely mathematically the probability of obtaining a particular result lying in the range $\bar{x} + N_1 s$ and $\bar{x} + N_2 s$.

The probability

$$P = \int_{N_1}^{N_2} \left(\frac{1}{\sqrt{2\pi}} e^{-\frac{1}{2}N^2} \right) dN$$

The graph of the function $\frac{1}{\sqrt{2\pi}} e^{-\frac{1}{2}N^2}$ against N indicates how N is related to dP/dN, the rate of change of P with respect to N (Fig. 51), and has a shape similar to the histogram relating the proportion of animals whose individual lethal doses lie in a particular range. If the range were narrow enough and the number of animals killed large enough, the width of the units making up the histogram would become very narrow and the picture would resemble the smooth curve obtained with the function. When the function is integrated between $N = -1$ and $N = +1$, it is found that P is 0·68 so there are roughly two chances in three of obtaining a result lying in this range and experimentally roughly two-thirds of the animals should have their individual lethal doses lying in this range. Integration between $N = -2$ and $N = +2$ gives a value of 0·955, and over 95 per cent of the animals would be expected to have their individual lethal doses lying within two standard deviation units of the mean.

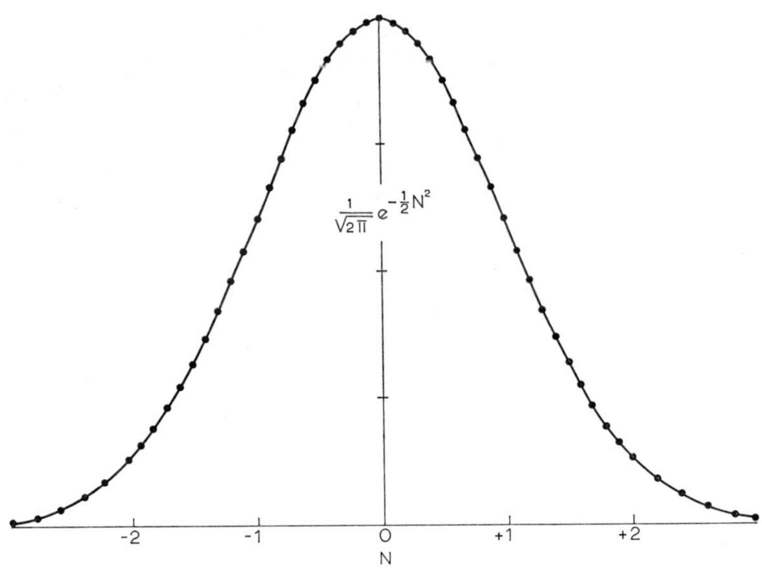

Fig. 51. Graph of P against N.

In practice it is tedious to measure individual lethal doses, it is much easier to give the same dose to a group of animals and observe the proportion of animals killed. This will include not only the animals for whom the chosen dose was the individual lethal dose but also all those whose individual lethal dose was less than this. This proportion should correspond to the probability of obtaining a result lying in the range from $N = -\infty$ up to the value for the chosen dose. If the dose were in fact the mean dose, $\bar{x}$, the upper limit would be $N = 0$ and the value of P would be 0·5. This dose $\bar{x}$ which experimentally kills 50 per cent of the animals is usually referred to as LD_{50}. The dose which is less than this by one standard deviation ($N = -1$) should kill just under 16 per cent of the animals, the dose one standard deviation above LD_{50} ($N = +1$) should kill just over 84 per cent (and $84 - 16 = 68$ per cent of the animals have individual lethal doses lying between $N = -1$ and $N = +1$). As the proportion of animals affected by the dose is related to N by the expression for normal distribution, it should be the same for a particular value of N for any drug provided the sensitivity to the drug is normally distributed. The relationship between the actual dose, x, producing effects in a proportion, p, of the animals, and N, the normal equivalent deviation corresponding to p, is given by the equation

$$x = \bar{x} \pm Ns$$

so the graph of x against N is a straight line from which $\bar{x}$ can be calculated. In practice it is usual to add 5 to the value of N so that all figures become positive and these are called probits. In experiments producing all-or-none responses, therefore, doses are given to groups of animals, and the dose is plotted against the probit of the percentage in the group which produce a response. It should be noted that the graph of dose against percentage is not linear.

Because there are reasons for believing that the distribution may be lognormal rather than normal it is probably more correct to plot log dose, rather than dose, against the probit of the percentage of the group which responds. Graph paper can be bought in which one axis is divided logarithmically and the other in probability units (Fig. 52) and so does away with the need for tables of logarithms and probits.

Toxicity tests

In designing a toxicity test it is desirable to arrange that in all about half the animals survive, in other words that the doses tested are distributed evenly about the mean. For example in a test of the oral toxicity of cytisine in mice the following results were obtained (Table III).

TABLE III

Dose μmoles/kg.	log dose	Mice killed		Probit	% expected from graph (E)	O − E	Contribution to chi²
		No.	% (O)				
208	2·318	0	3·5*		11	7·5	0·07
368	2·566	4/10	40	4·75	31 } N′	9	0·035
544	2·736	5/10	50	5·00	51 } N′	1	0
648	2·812	6/10	60	5·25	60 } N′	0	0
820	2·914	7/10	70	5·52	71 } N′	1	0
1005	3·002	8/10	80	5·84	80 } N′	0	0
1309	3·117	10/10	94·8*		83 } N′	11·8	0·07
							Total 0·175

* Total number killed 35/70; number of doses, $K = 7$; number of animals per dose $= 10$.

From the graph, $LD_{50} = 535$ μmoles/kg. (Fig. 52); there is actually no need to calculate the values of log dose and probit if the special log dose-probability graph paper is used.

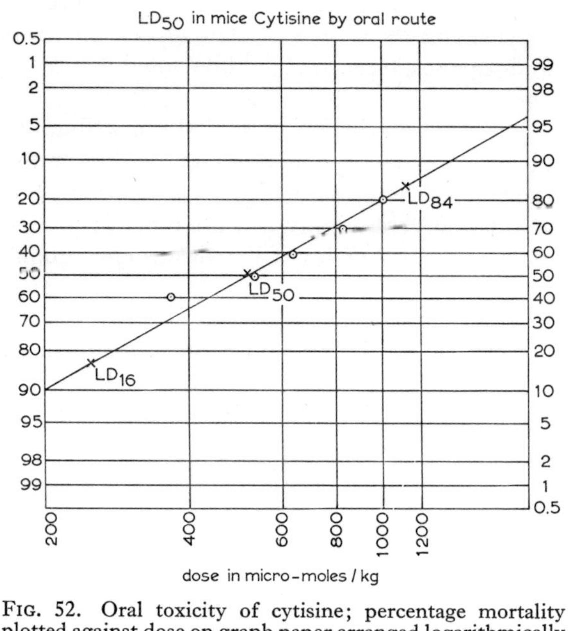

FIG. 52. Oral toxicity of cytisine; percentage mortality plotted against dose on graph paper arranged logarithmically along the x-axis and in probability units along the y-axis (L. J. McLeod, 1968, M.Sc. thesis, University of Edinburgh).

To calculate the fiducial limits of this estimate by the method of Litchfield and Wilcoxon[1], it is necessary to see how the results differ from the expected result, E, obtained from the graph. A correction must be made for results of 0 or 100 per cent, in these experiments only values of 0 or 10 per cent and 100 or 90 per cent would be obtainable with doses in this range. The values marked with an asterisk are obtained from a table relating the value, E, expected from the graph with the value likely to be obtained when the experimental value is 0 or 100 per cent. The difference between the observed (O) and expected (E) results is now used to assess the contribution to chi^2 from each sample, conveniently obtained from a nomogram relating E, $E-O$, and chi^2. The total contribution, i.e. the sum of the contributions from each sample (0·175) multiplied by the number of animals in each group (10), is then compared with the value of chi^2 for the particular number of degrees of freedom, which is (the number of dose-levels tested -2), i.e. 5. At a level of probability of $p = 0{\cdot}05$, this gives a value of chi^2 (from tables) of 11·1, which is greater than the observed value, 1·75, so the results are not significantly heterogeneous and the line is a good fit.

The graph is now used to calculate the dose effective in 16 per cent and in 84 per cent of the animals ($LD_{16} = 250$, $LD_{84} = 1122$ μmoles/kg.) and the slope function, S, is calculated;

$$S = \frac{LD_{84}/LD_{50} + LD_{50}/LD_{16}}{2} = 2{\cdot}11$$

The number of animals tested for which the expected effects lie between 16 and 84, N', is next calculated; this includes all those bracketed together in column E, i.e. 6 out of the 7 groups, so $N' = 60$.

The confidence limits of LD_{50} ($p = 0{\cdot}05$) are given by

$$f\,LD_{50} = S^{\left(\frac{2\cdot77}{\sqrt{N'}}\right)} = 2{\cdot}11^{\left(\frac{2\cdot77}{\sqrt{60}}\right)} = 2{\cdot}11^{0\cdot36} = 1{\cdot}3$$

The calculation is again simplified by the use of nomograms provided by Litchfield and Wilcoxon. The limits are therefore $535 \times 1{\cdot}3 = 696$ μmoles/kg. and $535 \div 1{\cdot}3 = 411$ μmoles/kg.

[1] Litchfield, J. T. & Wilcoxon, F. (1949). *J. Pharmac.*, **96**, 99.

Appendix II

MOLECULAR WEIGHTS OF DRUGS AND A GUIDE TO THEIR STABILITY IN SOLUTION

Values in parenthesis are the equivalent weights of compounds which contain 2 molecules of drug in each molecule of salt.

U. = Solutions last only for hours
S. = Solutions last for days
VS. = Solutions last for weeks
A. = Keep the stock solution acid (pH 4)
Asc. = Add ascorbic acid (see companion volume, p. 11)

Note. Some commercial solutions for injection marked with an asterisk (*) keep for much longer periods than solutions prepared from solids and water.

Drug	Mol. wt.	Stability
Acetazolamide	222·2	*S.*
sodium	244·2	
Acetylcholine chloride	181·7	*U.A.*
bromide	226·2	
iodide	273·1	
Acetyl-β-methylcholine (Methacholine)		
chloride	195·7	*U.A.*
bromide	240·2	
Acetylsalicylic acid (Aspirin)	180·2	
(solid *VS.*)		
Adrenaline	183·2	*U.A.Asc.*
hydrochloride	219·7	
hydrogen tartrate	333·3	
Amethocaine hydrochloride	300·8	*S.*
Amphetamine sulphate, B_2, H_2SO_4	368·5 (184·2)	*VS.*
Amylobarbitone sodium	248·3	*U.*
Apomorphine hydrochloride $\frac{1}{2}H_2O$	312·8	*VS.*
Atropine	289·4	*S.*
sulphate, B_2, H_2SO_4, H_2O	694·8 (347·4)	
Butyrylcholine chloride	209·7	*U.A.*
iodide	301·1	
Carbachol chloride	182·7	*U.A.*
Carbimazole	186·2	*U.*
(solid *VS.*)		
Chloralose	309·5	
(solid *VS.*)		

Chlordiazepoxide hydrochloride (Librium)	336·2	*S.*
Chlorpromazine hydrochloride	355·3	*VS.*
Choline chloride	139·6	*VS.*
Cinchocaine hydrochloride	379·9	*VS.*
Cocaine hydrochloride	339·8	*S.*
Codeine	317·4	*VS.*
hydrochloride, $2H_2O$	371·9	
sulphate, B_2, H_2SO_4, $3H_2O$	750·9 (375·5)	
Decamethonium iodide	512·0	*VS.*
'Dial' compound—diallylbarbituric acid and urethane*		*VS.*
Dimercaprol	124·2	*VS.*
dimercaprol injection, 5% w/v in arachis oil		
Dimethylphenylpiperazinium iodide (DMPP)	318·2	*VS.*
Ephedrine hydrochloride	201·7	*S.*
Ergotoxine ethane sulphonate	671·8	*VS.*
Ethanol	46	*S.*
Ether	74·12	*U.*
Ethylchloride (only used as vapour)	64·52	
Gallamine trietho-chloride	617·3	*VS.*
triethiodide	891·5	
Guanethidine sulphate, B_2, H_2SO_4	494·7 (247·3)	*S.*
Halothane (only used as vapour)	197·4	
Heparin sodium: solution for injection: usual strengths 1,000, 5,000, 10,000 and 20,000 units/ml., *VS.* when kept below 25°C. Solid heparin usually contains between 110 and 130 units/mg.		
Hexamethonium bromide	362·2	*VS.*
Hexobarbitone sodium	258·3	*U.*
Histamine di(hydrogen phosphate), B, $2H_3PO_4$	307·1	*U.A.*
Homatropine hydrobromide	356·3	*S.*
5-Hydroxytryptamine	176·1	*S.*
creatinine sulphate	405·4	
Isoprenaline	211·2	*U.A.Asc.*
hydrochloride	247·7	
sulphate, B_2, H_2SO_4, $2H_2O$	556·6 (278·3)	
Leptazol (for injection)*	138·2	*VS.*

Lignocaine hydrochloride, H_2O	288·8	*VS.*
Lobeline hydrochloride	373·9	*VS.*
Meprobamate	218·3	*S.*
Mersalyl sodium	505·9	*S.*
(for injection)* *VS.*		
Methadone hydrochloride	345·9	*VS.*
(–) Morphine hydrochloride, $3H_2O$	375·8	
Morphine sulphate, B_2, H_2SO_4, $5H_2O$	758·8 (379·4)	*VS.*
Nalorphine hydrobromide	392·3	*VS.*
Neostigmine bromide	303·2	*VS.*
methane sulphonate	334·3	
Nicotine	162·2	*VS.*
di (hydrogentartrate)		
B, (hydrogentartrate)$_2$, $2H_2O$	498·4	
Nikethamide	178·2	*S.*
(for injection)* *VS.*		
Noradrenaline	169·1	*U.A.Asc.*
hydrogentartrate, H_2O	337·3	
Ouabain	728·8	*VS.*
(Strophanthin G)		
Oxotremorine	206·3	*VS.*
Oxyphenonium bromide	428·4	*S.*
Pentobarbitone sodium	248·3	*S.*
('Nembutal' for injection, *VS.*)		
Pethidine hydrochloride	283·8	*S.*
(Meperidine hydrochloride)		
Phenadoxone hydrochloride	388·0	*VS.*
Phenazocine hydrobromide, B, HBr, $\frac{1}{2}H_2O$	411·4	*VS.*
Phenobarbitone sodium	254·2	*S.*
Phenoxybenzamine hydrochloride	340·3	*VS.*
(when neutralized to form the active species, *U.*)		
Phenytoin sodium	274·3	*VS.*
Physostigmine sulphate, B_2, H_2SO_4, H_2O	648·8 (324·4)	*U.A.*
salicylate	413·5	
Picrotoxin	602·6	*VS., A.*
Pilocarpine nitrate	271·3	*S.*
Posterior pituitary extract (vasopressin)		*U.A.*
Potassium chloride	74·6	*VS.*
Potassium iodide	166·0	*VS.*
Potassium perchlorate	138·6	*VS.*
Procaine hydrochloride	272·8	*S.*

Propionylcholine chloride	195·7	*U.A.*
iodide	287·1	
Propranolol hydrochloride	295·7	*S.*
Reserpine	608·7	*S.*
Sodium cyanide	49	*S.*
Sodium salicylate	160·1	*VS.*
Sulphacetamide sodium	254·2	*S.*
Suxamethonium chloride, $2H_2O$	397·4	
bromide, $2H_2O$	486·3	*U.*
iodide	544·2	
Thialbarbitone sodium	286·3	*U.*
Thiopentone sodium	264·3	*U.*
Theophylline	180·2	*VS.*
Thyroxine	776·9	*S.*
Triethylcholine iodide	146·2	*VS.*
(+) Tubocurarine chloride, $5H_2O$	785·8	*VS.*
Tyramine hydrochloride	173·6	*VS.*
Urethane	89·1	*S.*
Vasopressin	1,005	*U.A.*

ROBERT CUNNINGHAM AND SONS LTD, LONGBANK WORKS, ALVA

NOTES

NOTES

NOTES

NOTES

NOTES